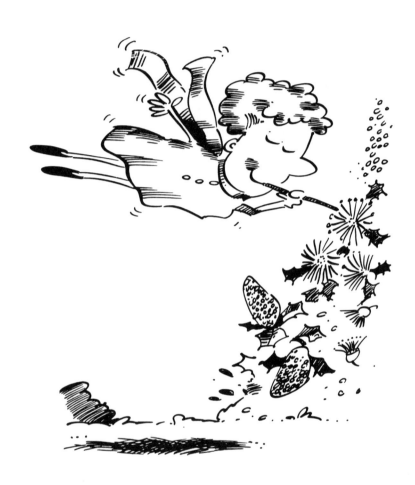

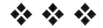

FIND YOUR NATURAL WEIGHT

The NECTAR *way*

Judith McFadden
with Jenny McFadden
Drawings by Gordon Bain

NOTICE!

Consult your health care provider or physician before using this book, especially if you have any medical or health conditions that prevent you from following the suggestions and exercises contained herein. Use your common sense. The publisher and authors are not responsible for any adverse effects or consequences resulting from using this book.

The Cover

The little Australian hummingbird, a New Holland Honeyeater, is sharing the nectar of a Banksia blossom with a bee. The Banksia species was named after Sir Joseph Banks, the botanist who accompanied Captain Cook on his voyage of the discovery of Australia. New Holland was the name given to Australia by Dutch explorers. ("New Holland Honeyeater" photograph by Michael Morocombe. Used by permission.)

ISBN 0-944337-24-4

Library of Congress Catalog Card Number: 94-68732

Printed in the United States of America

10 9 8 7 6 5 4 3 2

Quantity Purchases

Companies, professional groups, clubs and other organizations may qualify for special terms when ordering quantities of this title. For ordering information contact the Sales Department, New View Publications, P. O. Box 3021, Chapel Hill, NC 27515-3021. (919) 942-8491

Drawings by Gordon Bain.

Text design by Dixon J. Smith.

Cover design by Lizardesque, 17a Walton Crescent, Abbotsford, NSW, Australia.

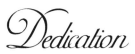

Dedication

To Helen

Acknowledgments

I would like to thank Dr. William Glasser, who helped me to understand his ideas about control theory and to apply them in my own life. Without control theory this book could not have been written. I also appreciate his faith in the Nectar Program.

Thanks to my husband, Max, who supports me so well, and to my three children, Jenny, Louise and Mark, who have all added their own particular talents and skills to this venture. Jenny took the journey with me and made a significant contribution to this book; Louise took time from a busy career to help organize our business; and Mark printed work of high quality when we needed it "yesterday." Together we have grown, and we have grown together.

Special Thanks

To Perry Good, who recognized the potential of Nectar to help many other people, and who in the process has become a friend.

To Marjorie Hudson, who edited this book. I was constantly impressed by her ability to clarify the message for the reader.

To Gordon Bain, whose cartoons add so much meaning to this book. He brought difficult concepts to life with warmth and humor.

To Dale Atrens for permission to use material from his book *Don't Diet* (Bantam 1988).

To Jenny, Robin, Jill, Ren, Edward and Cathy, members of the first experimental group, who had the faith to try the Nectar ideas.

To the participants of the pilot Nectar Program, who were prepared to risk their money as well as their bodies, and who gave us honest and rewarding evaluations.

To my reality therapy and control theory colleagues and the participants in the groups I have taught, who have contributed to my deeper understanding of Nectar.

And especially to Fred, Maria, Zika, Trevor and all the staff at New View who gave their friendship and support to an Aussie away from home.

Table of Contents

Preface

This book was written in answer to my search for a way of life that did not include *dieting*—the constant worry about the effect of food on weight, the constant self-denial, the constant concentration on food. The ideal world, I decided, would contain instead the freedom to eat whatever looked good, the belief that it was OK to be happy with one's appearance, and the knowledge that my body weight would remain constant without continual focus on food.

In my search for this ideal world, I looked closely at the relationship between eating, food, and weight, and began to define this relationship by its process, instead of by what it said on the scales. My study resulted in a personal journey that took me from the painful world of the long-term dieter into the quite pleasant world of the *natural eater*. I took this journey in the company of my daughter, Jenny, another long-term dieter. Together, we studied the behavior of both dieters and non-dieters and discovered a startling difference in one area only: the way they *think*.

My daughter and I gave up *dieting* and instead started experimenting with different ways of *thinking about food*. The journey we took was into unknown territory; many of the ideas we tried out were counter to society's traditional beliefs about weight, eating, and food. The decision to give up dieting was not so difficult, because so much of the literature affirmed that diets do not work. The hard part was learning how to change our thinking about eating. This was the step that had been missing in all the material we studied.

The Nectar Groups

To expand our study, we formed a small support group, sharing and discussing their new ideas with others. The group format was so helpful to members that I became convinced such groups could help others as well. Thus was born the Nectar program, a series of small groups led by trained instructors to help dieters learn to give up dieting and become natural eaters. Many former dieters in Australia, and now in the United States, have used this process to help them feel free, happy, confident, and in control around food—and in the rest of their lives as well. For more information about the Nectar groups, refer to the addendum in the back of this book.

How This Book Evolved

The Nectar program uses the ideas of Nectar and control theory, and puts them into practice in small groups, resulting in an effective learning process. I observed that Nectar ideas alone, so very different from the conventional wisdom of dieting, seemed a powerful tool for some. I realized that a book explaining my ideas might be a good way for others to get started with the job of giving up dieting and changing their lives.

This book focuses on providing useful ideas and exercises to help dieters learn on their own how to give up dieting. *The Nectar Way* emphasizes the positive, offers tips on making decisions, feeling satisfied, and taking charge of your eating by understanding how your mind and body work. The negative thinking and guilt associated with restrictive dieting goes out the window—along with restrictive diets. Your natural abilities to nurture yourself emerge as you begin to think about eating in an entirely new way.

How To Use This Book

Read it through once to get the whole range of useful ideas and how they fit together. This book will give you positive energy to try some new things! When you're done, go back to Chapters 6–11 and read a chapter a week, trying out the ideas one by one. Go to restaurants, eat with friends, eat alone, and try the exercises. As you do so, the new concepts will begin to take hold and shape a whole new pattern of eating behavior. It takes time, but as you get used to thinking about food in new ways, you may feel so good that you'll never want to go back to dieting.

If you find control theory useful in shaping your eating habits, you might want to do some further reading about it. Control theory can be applied in many ways to help you shape various aspects of your life. *In Pursuit of Happiness*, by E. Perry Good, is a good book to start with. Others are listed in the back of this book.

Chapter 1

THE NECTAR WAY

This is a book about freedom. Freedom from the tyranny of diets and weighing yourself, freedom from the fear of putting on weight, freedom from the anxiety associated with binge eating, freedom from the feeling of being controlled by food. Imagine being free to choose and enjoy whatever food you want to eat from whatever is at hand, free to feel good about yourself, free to allow your body to assume its natural weight. This is what it's like to be a natural eater.

Sounds like dieters' heaven? Only to be experienced after you die, if you've been "good?" Two years ago I would have agreed with you. Believing that the only way to get thin was to restrict how much food I ate, I assumed then that the only way to lose weight was to diet. I have since learned there is another way. What I have learned these past two years has given me freedom that I did not believe was possible. I have learned to behave like a natural eater. I, and many other people who have learned these ideas, now live a more peaceful, pleasant life where food is no longer a major focus. Instead, it is just something to be enjoyed when we are ready for it, to enhance our pleasure without dominating our lives.

Reaching this pleasant state was not painful, and did not require willpower or self-denial. The new behaviors I learned were so much more comfortable than the old dieting behaviors that it has been simple to establish them as a new way of life—what I call *The Nectar Way*.

What Is The Nectar Way?

The Nectar Way is not a diet. It is a way of thinking, feeling, choosing, and acting in relation to food. It is a way of focusing your attention on serving your needs, and a way of balancing and evaluating conflicting needs and desires to best serve you. In reading this book, you will discover some new concepts about how your mind and body work. Some of them are radical ideas for dieters! These concepts sometimes go against conventional wisdom, but they are not hard to understand and are extremely useful. You will learn why modern nutritionists say diets don't work—and why natural eating does.

NECTAR Stands For Natural Eating, Control Theory, And Results

Nectar teaches specific new skills that will help you make the transition to becoming a natural eater. Many of the new concepts you will learn are based on control theory, a recognized modern theory of human psychology that has been used for many years to help people focus on meeting their own needs. I have included in this book a primer on control theory to help you grasp the underlying basics of Nectar. The Nectar Way is based on thinking and understanding how your mind and body work. Once you understand these things, you won't be surprised that diets don't work. Most of what our culture believes about eating is way off base. The results you will get from the Nectar Way are slow, long-term, and a permanent part of your life!

Along the way, you will find several examples of the kinds of human dilemmas people face when they are giving up dieting forever and becoming natural eaters. From "What will my mother say?" to "How do I convince my waiter that I really *do* want dessert first?", questions and concerns will be answered thoroughly with suggestions and examples of how others have faced such problems. You will learn that you can do crazy-sounding things such as eat all the chocolate you want—as long as it's *you* making the decision and not the chocolate. You will learn how to use an extraordinary new freedom to eat what you want and choose what makes you feel satisfied. You will learn how to live in the *pleasant present.* What better time than now?

Chapter 2

JENNY'S STORY

I want to tell you that I have lost weight. I don't know how much, and actually that isn't important to me anymore. I was a size 20-22 when I started to learn about Nectar eighteen months ago. Now I'm about a size 16, so it has been a gradual change. The weight I lost went away without dieting, and I still eat everything I enjoy. I don't count calories and I don't weigh myself. I listen to my body in a natural way, just like when I was a child.

Before Nectar, I had dieted for eighteen years, starting when I was about fourteen. I tried every program you can imagine. They told me I had to have willpower over food. What I learned was this: to look the way you want to look, you need to control your eating. I now know the calorie count of every food you can name, what portions I should eat each day, the cholesterol count—you name it. But it didn't help my weight problem. The more I learned, the less it helped. And when I lost weight (which I did, in varying amounts), I still felt fat inside. For example, I remember one experience I had when I was teaching at a secondary school. I was a size 12 then, and one day some boys told me, "You look really nice, Miss." I thought to myself, "No, I'm fat." I told them this and they looked at me in disbelief. That was the crazy thinking I had learned.

The problem was, the more I dieted, the more I was preoccupied with food, constantly thinking about food, planning what I could or could not have, criticizing myself when I ate forbidden foods, still worried that people thought I was fat. I still believed that to be acceptable, successful, and attractive, I should be thinner. I lived in the future, telling myself, "I need to be thinner before I buy any more clothes," "I have to be thinner before I go dancing, or swimming, or wear jeans." I felt very unhappy and unfulfilled, and I wasted a lot of time and energy in a negative way. These same thoughts and beliefs made me fat again, time after time.

It isn't until you change the way you think about food and about yourself that you will be able to lose weight permanently. You will feel anxious, guilty, unhappy, and deprived if your mind is stuck thinking thoughts such as: "I feel fat," "I need to be thinner and then life will be better," "I shouldn't eat forbidden foods," "I can't swim in public because people will think I'm fat." You will eat to take care of yourself and to make yourself feel better.

We have been told for so long that *food* is our problem, that we need more willpower over food, that we need to restrict our food, count calories, eat only the prescribed foods on the list, use diet tablets, drink replacement meals, eat only fruit for breakfast, combine certain foods, eat no fat—the list goes on.

If any of these were successful, why is there a billion-dollar weight-loss industry? Much of the advice given by diet programs is well intentioned. For example, less fat in your diet *is* healthy. The problem lies in the fact that we need to feel free to choose these foods because we *want* to—we *choose* to—not because of a diet restriction that immediately leaves us feeling deprived. We dieters have been putting the cart before the horse. We have been thinking that to be thinner means to be happier about ourselves. So we diet to be thinner. Actually, we need to feel happier about ourselves to be thinner!

Question: How do you become happy?

Answer: I have become a happier person and my happiness seems almost completely independent of my weight! I'm happy because I have a new freedom to:

- Live now and feel good about myself
- Enjoy all foods without guilt
- Give control of my weight over to my body
- Never diet again, feel deprived, or worry about food and weight

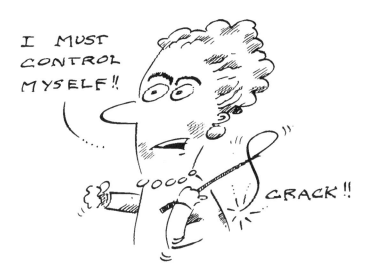

Question:

What should I do now that is different? What helps me to lose weight?

Answer:

I feel good about me, without undue self-criticism.

- I listen to my body.
- I eat when I am hungry (a fantastic experience—very satisfying and pleasurable).
- I feel happy about leaving food on the plate, or even turn down a favorite food because I am full.
- I eat foods that are the *best* (in quality, taste etc.), leaving inferior foods and treating my body to only the best.

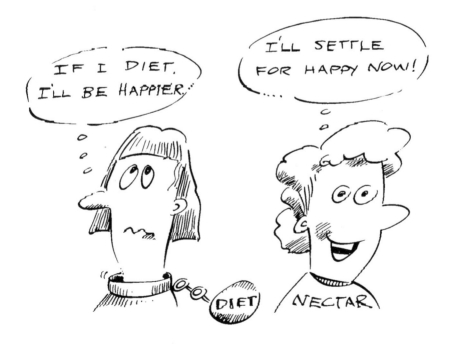

- I recognize that I have different ways I can deal with emotional hunger, rather than using food to take care of myself.

In the long term, you can judge that my intake of food is less than before, but not because I'm trying to lose weight. Instead, I am giving my body food on demand. In turn, my bingeing or overeating becomes less and less because I feel positive about food, and I eat only quality foods, really enjoying them. Most of all, I have learned the thought processes that support my new behaviors.

Once upon a time, a smorgasbord was an excuse to allow myself to eat everything in sight. I call it being a *tourist eater*. The tourist eater thinks, "I'd better eat everything because I won't be back here again (I'll be on a diet again)." Now, I find that I don't *really* like one of the big smorgasbord restaurants I went to because the quality isn't good enough. The last time I went, I can honestly say I found only the potato skins, some fresh vegetables, and the bread even worth trying. I sampled a few other things, and found them to be *not good enough*. It was a real shock to my system to walk out having eaten only a handful of food and think, "I'll go somewhere else for a better quality experience next time."

My Quality World Is Now

My future now seems very different from the one I imagined years ago, and here are several reasons for this.

I have power in my world. I now have confidence that my weight will never rise again. I feel much more happy about the way I look, the way I feel about myself, and I am comfortable about me for the first time in my life. I never felt comfortable before, even when I was at my thinnest.

I have fun with food and my body enjoys it too. I love food, and now I enjoy everything without guilt. I make the choices about what I will have and I listen to my body. My body is talking to me again. I now understand how a natural eater thinks, and I understand how I can turn down chocolate mud cake sometimes because I really don't want it, not because I feel deprived. It is a pleasant present indeed.

My body feels "right" for right now. I may be thinner the next time you see me, or I might not. At this point I feel comfortable with myself. My natural weight might be around this size. Actually, I think I might get smaller very gradually. I know the choice will be mine from here.

I know how to eat naturally for life. I now have the tools and techniques that I know work, and I am still learning and practicing them the same as if I were learning a new language. And the new language is fantastic— it's the language of freedom.

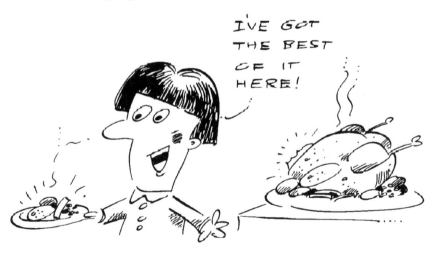

Freedom, fun, love, and power—you can have it all!

I am sure you've noticed my enthusiasm. It shows on the outside as well. A new way of thinking has helped me feed and balance *all* my needs. I feel great, and it is *my* opinion that counts most in how I feel about myself! Here are some experiences that I predict you, too, will have if you learn Nectar thinking:

- You will leave food on the plate (and feel good about it) because you have had enough.
- You will find yourself looking forward to being hungry because you know something tasty will be waiting.
- You will want to wait to eat until you are hungry because you enjoy it so much.
- You will turn down previously unforgettable food because you discover that it wasn't really all that great—it just used to be forbidden.
- You will find an opened packet of your favorite cookies that you forgot about.
- You will go out to dinner and find yourself choosing only the best foods because you can have whatever you like.
- You will notice that you haven't overeaten or binged for a while when it used to happen every other day.
- You will feel in control of your life, be more assertive towards food, have more fun and feel good about yourself.

Nectar can change your life. I know, because it has changed mine and the lives of so many people I have seen go through the Nectar training program.

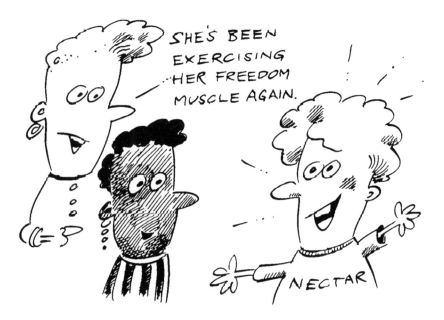

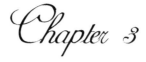

Chapter 3

NATURAL EATING VS. DIETING

How did we end up in an endless diet?

Ask yourself this question: "In relation to food, have I been *good* today?" If you are a dieter, I can almost guarantee your answer was something like this: "What about that sugar I put on my breakfast cereal?" or "Oh, no, I did have some chocolate but that was yesterday," or "I shouldn't have put that cream in my coffee," or "I was so good last weekend!" Whether you *were* "good" or "bad," you are certainly preoccupied with how good or bad you've been. This is the first sign of an unnatural eater.

The Unnatural Eater

Whether you are fat or thin, you feel restricted and uncomfortable around food because you eat it for reasons that have very little to do with the main reason all animal species were born with mouths and stomachs—to be able to nourish ourselves and stay alive! I use the term "unnatural" because it *cannot* be natural to spend your life feeling restricted and uncomfortable about eating, which is, after all, a necessary process.

Some people manage to live with the discomfort and lack of freedom of unnatural eating and keep their appearance at a level acceptable to them; others go on and off diets, lose weight and regain it, constantly criticizing themselves for their lack of willpower. On the outside, unnatural eaters may come in all shapes and sizes, but on the inside, we all go through the same uncomfortable feelings and thoughts. It doesn't have to be this way!

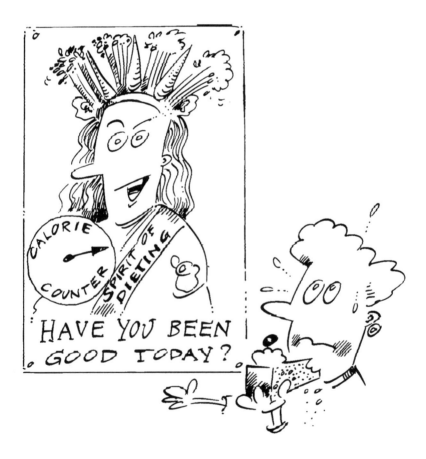

The Natural Eater

Believe it or not, there is a group of people who think, "What does being good have to do with food? That's a stupid question!" They might then have thought, "Well, have I eaten healthy things today—did I eat any junk food?" For these people, food is simply there to be enjoyed if they need it. It is neither good nor bad. Eating is no more important than all the other experiences they have in their lives. These people are *natural eaters.* For them, food and eating are necessary to stay alive and provide nourishment. Probably, most natural eaters would not have picked up this book in the first place because eating, food, and weight are simply not problems for them.

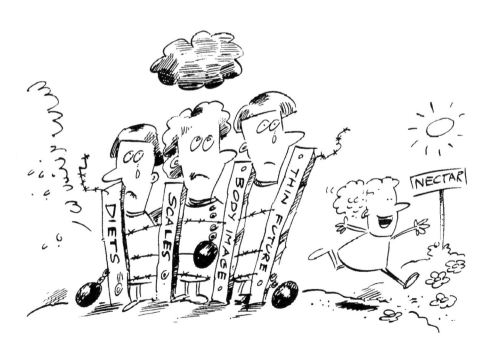

How Is An Unnatural Eater Different From A Natural Eater?

It's all in the way you think! Let me give you an example. I am an unnatural eater, and my father was a natural eater. I used to stay with him one night a week when he was in his early nineties and still living alone—I would do his shopping and keep him company. He didn't get out much, and I used to make sure that one pleasure he had was good things to eat. He was particularly fond of a brand of fancy chocolates, so each week I would make sure that he had a supply of them (a box with about 16 pieces in it). After dinner, he might say, "I think I would like something sweet—could you bring me one of those chocolates?" I would get one for him and take one for myself, depending on whether I was on or off a diet at the time.

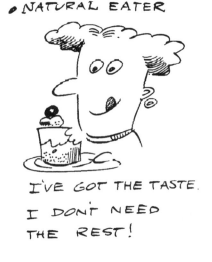

NATURAL EATER

I'VE GOT THE TASTE. I DON'T NEED THE REST!

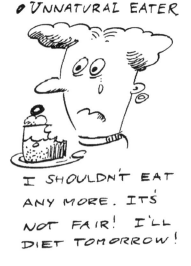

UNNATURAL EATER

I SHOULDN'T EAT ANY MORE. IT'S NOT FAIR! I'LL DIET TOMORROW!

What happened next may make you groan in recognition. He would go to bed early, and I would sit there in front of the TV, mooning about those chocolates, wanting to eat one (one? more likely the whole box!) and knowing that I should leave them for him. They would almost burn a hole in the refrigerator. One night (with what I thought was great restraint) I ate two, and the next week he complained, "All of my chocolates are gone!" Each week I would torture myself about those chocolates, and usually I would look for other, less satisfying things to eat instead. I would even buy substitute foods like cupcakes and hide them to eat after he went to bed. I came to dread the nights alone there. I "escaped" by going to the movies, calling friends, or anything else to get those chocolates out of my mind. Whether I was "good" or "not good," whether I gobbled up those chocolates or left them alone, I was an unnatural eater. My mind was absorbed, completely and unnaturally, in the subject of eating.

Next is the worst part. The following week I checked out his refrigerator and discovered that my father had eaten only about two or three of those chocolates—not even one a day! It struck me that those darn chocolates had much less importance for him than they did for me. I didn't know how he did it, but I wished I could be that way, able to have enticing food in the house, and to think of it as just something that was available but not "talking to me." I wanted to be able to choose freely between foods, so that sometimes I would actually prefer a carrot or a piece of celery to one of those chocolates. To feel secure enough to have chocolates in the house, and to have the freedom within myself to choose not to eat them—those were my goals.

My search for that feeling of security and freedom is the subject of this book. These days, I have some of those same chocolates in my bedside drawer, almost as a talisman. I can feel satisfied with one, and a box lasts me a long time because I don't always think of eating one. The thought that comes to mind quite often, which I still find almost unbelievable, is "No, they're a bit too sweet." How did I change?

I changed my thinking. The difference between a natural and an unnatural eater is in the way you think in relation to food, both the way you process information about the food itself and your behavior towards it.

Natural eaters expect to remain at their natural weight without worrying about what or how much they eat. They eat what their bodies need, rather than what they think they should, and they know that it is quite normal and natural to leave any food that is in excess of their requirements. They are not fanatical about this. If something they really enjoy is available, they might eat more than they need. However, instead of making a resolution to be good tomorrow, they listen to the signals their body gives them to decide how much they need.

Unnatural eaters, on the other hand, put themselves through a lot of unnecessary pain because of what they have learned as dieters. They are afraid of gaining weight and they expect their bodies to get fat. They consider what they eat, they worry about its effect on their weight, they do their best to control themselves, and many of them spend a lot of time criticizing themselves for being overweight, having no willpower, and focusing on food in an effort to gain control.

The main difference between these two groups of people is in their thought patterns about food, weight, and eating. Unnatural eaters come in all shapes, sizes, ages, and sexes, and have chosen many different ways to attempt to gain control over their weight. The ideas in this book have helped people who are young, old, and in-between, male and female, whose unnatural eating behaviors may or may not be visible to other people as fat. They are people who predict that what they eat will make them fat, and see eating as a behavior to be controlled, whether they choose to control it or not.

So this is a book about behavior, not about food. There is no dieting, no restriction on what you can eat. There will be no gimmicky explanations of negative-calorie foods or food combinations, no special complements to your diet. You will look at the difference in the behaviors of a natural eater compared with those of a dieter or unnatural eater, and learn how to switch over from the behaviors that are making your life a misery.

You will develop a new lifestyle, one that fits with your own preferences about when, what, and how much to eat, what exercise you want to do, and how you want to live your life. You will feel comfortable around food, and able to make satisfying choices of behavior towards it. People who are already natural eaters will wonder what the fuss is about. They will say, "But that's what I do all the time!"

The information you learn here will provide you with an opportunity to find a freedom and peace of mind around food that you never thought possible. It takes work, in the form of memory, concentration, and practice, but you can become a person without a weight problem. You will feel free and satisfied around food, able to eat whatever you want without worrying about your weight. Instead of focusing on how people with weight problems behave, I have looked at the behaviors that natural eaters use and discovered the difference in their behavioral patterns, particularly their thinking and beliefs. I have showed you that I was an unnatural eater. Let me tell you my story and how I changed my life.

A Dieter's Profile

I have a forty-year history of problems with my weight: fat as a child and teenager, then many instances of losing and gaining weight during my adult life. I am a good dieter when I put my mind to it. I can stick to a diet program well, and have reached weight goals with several of the big weight-loss companies. (I even did it all by myself the first time, and wrote myself up in a women's magazine that had published their "Best-Ever Diet"; today it would be criticized for its cholesterol content!) While I am on the diet, I feel good about myself. The problems come when the diet is over. For a while I am able to restrict what I eat, but eventually I get tired of the restrictions and break out. Then all of the weight goes back, sometimes slowly, sometimes quickly, but inevitably.

I would feel discouraged, out of control, and unwilling to try again. There is always pain associated with dieting and it takes me a long time to make another commitment to losing weight. I would get a sinking feeling, thinking that "If I have to live the rest of my life restricting myself, feeling hungry and deprived around food, then life will not be worth living, so I might as well be fat!"

I really believed that my body did not burn up food the way other "normal" people's bodies did, and if I wanted to have a normal body I would have to settle for being hungry most of the time. I tried every dieter's trick in the book, but all I ended up with was the idea that there must be something wrong with me. This is the current thinking on weight loss: most people believe that

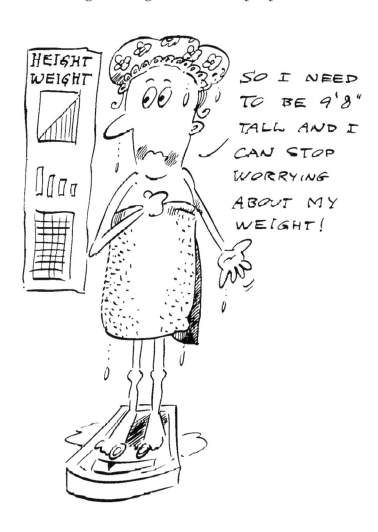

with all the knowledge we have, losing weight should be simple—there is something wrong with people who can't do it. But that is just not true.

What Is Wrong With Me?

The conventional explanation that society gives to unnatural eaters is that they are "eating away" at their problems. This implies that we are in some way lesser people than natural eaters—we have less willpower, we are more stupid, or we have bigger problems. I would sit in the car chewing away at something I had bought, thinking, "What's wrong with me? Why am I doing this? I don't feel good after I eat all this! What problems do I have? Why can't I stop?"

People with the problem of unnatural eating do not have different or more significant problems, or less willpower than others. Many of us do not have a metabolic problem, or a hypoglycemic problem, or any of the other things that we have looked at as explanations for being overweight. Also, we are not second-class citizens with lesser abilities because we are fat! In fact, frequent dieters are up against frightful odds that might daunt ordinary people. Research proves that when we diet, we have only a 5% chance of achieving permanent weight loss. Our bodies actually resist change, and when we limit what we eat to starvation level, they conserve every calorie we give them. Thus, dieters can get fat on less food than natural eaters eat to stay alive! What we have is a set of behaviors that we developed in order to lose weight, which are actually helping us to retain our weight problem.

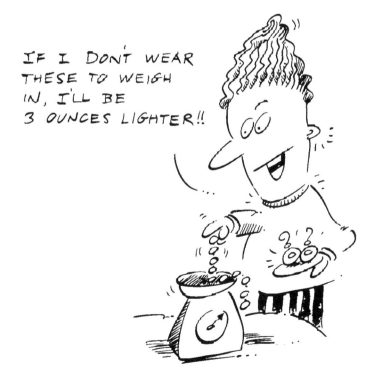

Chapter 4

DIETS DON'T WORK!

Dale Atrens, Ph.D., a psychobiologist at the University of Sydney, has done extensive research into the realities of dieting and weight loss, funded by the largest life sciences grant ever made by the Australian Research Grants Committee. After finding out what research said about dieting, he published a book entitled *Don't Diet* (New York: Bantam, 1988). His conclusions are:

- Fatness is not due to overeating or underexercise.
- Fatness alone does not cause early heart disease, cancer or early death.
- There is no single diet that is truly effective. If there were, there wouldn't be so many different diets on the market.
- For 95% of the population, it is impossible to lose significant amounts of weight and maintain the loss.
- The body's own metabolic rate, plus other hereditary and physiological reasons, are the determining factors in body size and shape.

Our culture demands of women that, in order to be considered beautiful, they pursue insane goals of slenderness. This pursuit often compromises not only their reproductive abilities, but their health and happiness as well. Men do not need to enforce compliance of the absurd code they have generated. Women are far better at policing themselves than anyone else could ever be.

Atrens' message is to give up dieting, eat sensibly, exercise moderately, and be satisfied with your body the way it is. Nectar simply adds to this message: think right, learn your new thoughts and beliefs, and you will eventually have it all—a healthy body, enjoyment of food in its place, and through control theory, the tools for making your life the way you want it to be.

By now, you can see there is nothing innately wrong with us unnatural eaters. All we have is a set of behaviors, probably developed over a long period of time, that are holding us in the diet mode. We probably got into this state because we were doing our best to look after ourselves—trying to get our bodies to be at what we believed was a healthy weight. Some of these behaviors we developed as children, some have come from dieting, and some from all the information we have absorbed from society. If you learned these behaviors, then you can learn other, more effective behaviors to replace them. One major difficulty with dieting is that we try for an absence of behavior to stop ourselves from eating. The message we give ourselves is, "You shouldn't eat that!" All we are doing is reminding ourselves that we want to eat, so that often we let go and eat when we don't need to.

Why Diets Don't Work

The most important reason why dieting only works for a while is that it severely limits our freedom. We are told what, how much, and when to eat. Someone works out for us what we should have, and we follow those instructions. Or we do it for ourselves, and limit our own freedom. Lack of freedom sets up feelings of anxiety. What do unnatural eaters do to feel better? They eat! So, the loss of freedom creates an endless cycle.

Diets also promote eating according to a schedule, which has nothing to do with the real reason why we should be eating—to nourish our bodies when they are hungry. When we diet, we learn to eat everything we are permitted to have, at designated times ("three meals and two snacks" as one diet company puts it). We are eating by the clock, whether we are hungry or not, and also learning not to leave a crumb of the food, whether we need it all or not, and whether we are enjoying it or not. We are teaching our brains to ignore hunger signals! If we become hungry an hour before a meal, we put up with the hunger, or do something to help ourselves "forget about it," such as go for a walk, drink some water, eat some carrot sticks, or anything else to take away the signal. As soon as we finish one meal, we look ahead on the diet chart to what we can have for the next one and the one after that, and the next day. . . .

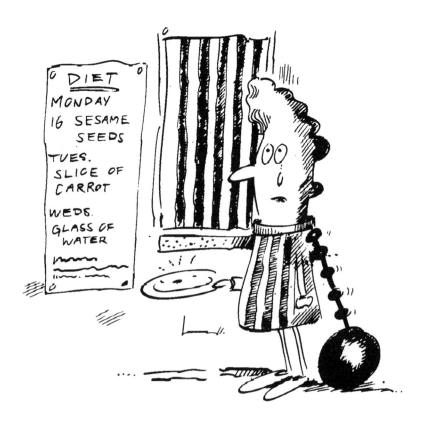

This means that, over time, we are training ourselves to ignore the signals our bodies used to give us: hunger and satisfaction. The signals are still coming to the brain, but the brain learns not to interpret them. These are the signals natural eaters rely on to balance their food intake with their body needs. If we can no longer rely on signals from the body we are nourishing, we begin to eat for reasons that are disconnected from our bodies' needs:

- It's lunch time or dinner time.
- Someone offers us something.
- Something looks good to eat.
- We are feeling lonely, angry, unhappy, bored.
- We have arrived home.
- We see an advertisement on TV.
- We ordered it.
- Our Mom made it for us.
- We are with a friend.

We eat for many reasons that really do not have much to do with whether we are hungry. Sometimes we eat even when we know we can't possibly be hungry, and go so far that we feel bloated and uncomfortable. Sometimes we are good for a period of time, then something seems to trigger us and we gobble everything in sight whether we enjoy it or not. When we go to smorgasbords, we eat much more than we need because it is available and we paid for it.

What Dieting Teaches Us

What dieting teaches us is to eat all of whatever we are allowed to eat, at times when we may or may not be hungry, and to ignore our hunger signals if they come at inappropriate times. This works while we are on the diet, but when we stop dieting, we then have no accurate reference points for knowing when to start and when to slow down in our eating. We always know what to eat when we stop dieting—all those things that were forbidden!

It is interesting to note that over the last half century, the proportion of overweight people in developed countries is higher than it has ever been, despite all the information that we now have about the number of calories in food, height-weight ratios, how to measure body fat, how much we weigh on our bathroom scales, which foods are high in fiber, fat, or cholesterol (a word most of us had not even heard until the seventies). Why, when we have so much information, are so many of us unnatural eaters? The answer is, the information itself is causing a lot of the problems. The more we know, the worse we feel! Now, why in the world is *that*?

Information As Criticism

I believe that all the information we now have about food, eating, and health has introduced additional problems into our eating habits. Knowing about calories, cholesterol, fat and salt content, carbohydrates simple and complex, vitamins (I could go on forever) has created a whole new minefield in deciding what to eat. There seems to be nothing that is truly safe to eat—even water has its problems! What the information has done is to set up double messages in our thinking about almost everything we eat: food is both tasty and nasty at the same time. It can be enticing but deadly, or legal but dull. We categorize it into good and bad. As soon as we put labels of this kind on food, we add an emotional element into choosing what to eat, and food assumes a higher importance in our lives than is necessary. And once again we are putting limits on what we eat and reducing our freedom.

On top of this, the information we get from our scales every day when we weigh ourselves is a source of criticism. In the old days, scales were not so readily available, and people relied on the fit of their clothes to tell them whether their weight had varied. Now, many people allow their scales to determine what sort of day they will have, and even how much they should eat, completely ignoring what their bodies might be telling them about whether they are hungry or not.

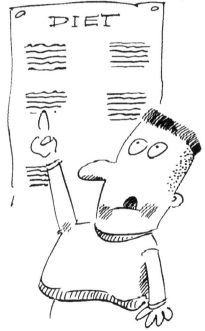

Criticism always breeds discomfort. Unfortunately for the dieter, discomfort is often a trigger for finding comfort, and an unnatural eater has learned the behavior of seeking food in order to feel more comfortable. This is why, when we are a few pounds overweight and make a resolution to eat less that day, the good resolution lasts only a

FOR DINNER THE DAY AFTER TOMORROW.. I CAN HAVE ......

couple of hours. Then we eat something for comfort and say to ourselves, "Well, I've blown it for another day—might as well eat whatever I want and start again tomorrow!" On the other hand, if we find we have lost a little weight, we have the perfect excuse for eating a little more that day. So when we weigh ourselves, we end up going around in circles without ever learning appropriate eating habits. It cannot be natural to have to live this way. People were not made to starve themselves or to diet. Read on—your life around food may never be the same again!

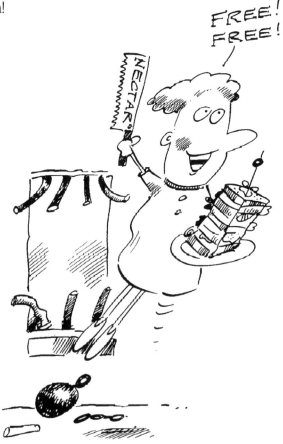

Chapter 5

A CONTROL THEORY PRIMER

The use of control theory in psychology originated with William Powers and was adapted by the renowned psychiatrist, William Glasser. I studied control theory as part of my basic training in reality therapy. After years of study and even more years of dieting, I realized how useful control theory could be in teaching new behaviors to chronic dieters. I'll give you the basics of control theory that you will need to change the way you think about food. These ideas will be very useful to you as you progress through learning the Six Principles of Nectar in the next six chapters. And you may find you can use these concepts in the rest of your life as well.

The control theory ideas we will use are based on the following principles. Each of these concepts relates to the process of making decisions, and making decisions about eating is the most important process in Nectar.

We are responsible for our own behavior, and what we choose to do is always something we can control. Often, when we are bingeing, we *feel* out of control. But the food is not making us eat it. We have, consciously or unconsciously, made a choice. Our job is to be sure our decisions are really based on our needs and desires.

We make choices to satisfy our needs. Our five basic needs are survival, power, love, fun, and freedom.

We get the information we need about the world through a set of "filters." Our three filters are senses, knowledge, and values.

Each of us has a "quality world." Our quality world is a collection of our ideals about how things should be: how we should be, look and behave.

Each of us has access to "signals" that tell us to do something. Signals occur when there is a gap between what we desire in our quality world and what we see happening. If we look in the mirror and we don't like what we see, we get a signal!

We must do something when we receive a signal, but we have options! Signals are powerful forces that generate behavior. But *we* get to choose what to do, and our behavior can consist of action, thoughts, feelings, and physiological changes all at the same time.

THE FIVE BASIC NEEDS

Control theory teaches that all human beings choose their behaviors in order to satisfy their five basic needs.

Survival

Everyone has a need to survive physically—as an individual and as a species. We feed ourselves, build shelters, pay mortgages, and plan for our physical safety to satisfy this need to survive. We can't give up eating altogether, as we need to eat to survive. This means we are continually faced with choices: how much, what, and when to eat. We make these choices all day long.

Love and Belonging

This is the need to love and be loved, to give, to be accepted for who you are, to trust, and to belong. We *need* to be loved. Without love, we would not survive.

Power and Recognition

We need to know that we matter, that what we do and who we are counts. Some people fulfill this need by seeking power over other people and things. Others satisfy the need by using their power to accomplish tasks. Others seek a sense of personal power to feel in control of their own lives. Whenever people feel out of control about eating, their power needs are frustrated. If you criticize yourself for eating or for your appearance, you tend to feel powerless.

Fun

Yes! You *need* to have fun. This is my personal favorite. When have you ever seen a diet that included this? If we are to lead a balanced life, we must satisfy our need for fun. It is important to our health and well-being, and it helps us satisfy our other needs as well. We are satisfying our need for fun when we enjoy the company of other people, spend time on a hobby, or taste some of our favorite food!

Freedom

We need to have freedom to choose what we do, where we go, and what we eat. Diets restrict freedom in all these areas. Nectar teaches that we choose freely what, when, and how much we eat, according to the individual needs of our bodies.

EATING AND THE FIVE BASIC NEEDS

If you sit and think about it, you will realize that *eating* fulfills all the five basic needs. If we eat when we are hungry, we know we will *survive*. When your mother makes you a special dinner for your birthday, you feel *loved*. When you decide to eat a candy bar (or *not* to eat a candy bar), you may feel *powerful*. When you pick out your favorite Italian food in a restaurant, you may be having *fun*. Whenever you make any choice about what to eat, you are exercising your *freedom*.

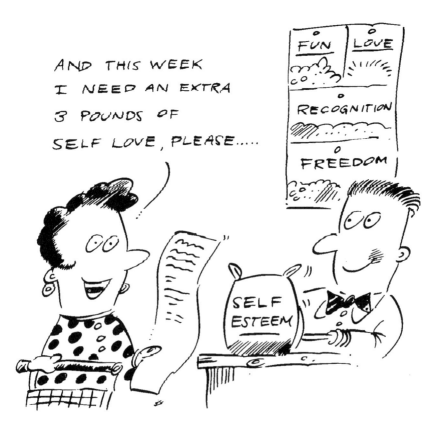

DIETS AND THE FIVE BASIC NEEDS

Survival

Most diets conform to certain standards of nutrition so that we will eat "properly." However, diets do limit our energy intake to less than our bodies actually require, so that we will burn up excess fat. There are two problems here. One is that the most available form of energy is the glycogen stored in our blood and our muscles. This is why after a few days on a very low-calorie diet, we start to run out of steam. The other problem is that our bodies do not like to be deprived of nourishment, and on a prolonged diet will go into "famine mode" by slowing down our metabolic rate to keep us alive. Our bodies' own *survival* mechanism has kicked in, and causes us to store as fat calories we need for energy.

Power

When we break a diet or feel bad about our weight, we criticize ourselves for our lack of willpower. We feel bad about our appearance. We tell ourselves we look awful. We are undermining our *power*. We may do well on a diet for a period of time, feeling powerful and in control as we get on the scale and it shows lost pounds. But because a diet can't serve our need for freedom, we are destined to end up frustrated.

Freedom

When we stay on a diet, we don't get to choose when, what, or how much we eat. We restrict ourselves in many ways, frustrating our need for *freedom*.

Fun

When we're on a diet and we can't eat our favorite food, or enjoy a dinner prepared by our best friend it's definitely not *fun*!

Love

You may feel awful telling your mother you can't enjoy her birthday cake, even if it symbolizes to her how much you *love* her.

So, dieting does not serve the five basic needs well at all. In fact, diets, for however long they may be successful, end up frustrating most, if not all, of your needs so greatly that going *off* a diet feels like the only alternative. You need to have the freedom to make your own choices.

THE THREE FILTERS

Senses

We can obtain information about the world only through our senses of sight, hearing, touch, taste and smell. If we can't see or hear well, our world differs from that of someone who can.

Knowledge

We filter new information through what we already know in order to make sense of it. If you know German, you'll be able to make sense of the street signs in Berlin. If you don't know Thai, good luck getting around Bangkok!

Values

Once we have made sense of the information, we decide whether we like it, dislike it, or feel neutral about it, according to our own personal values.

ALL-WE-KNOW WORLD

In the process of filtering all the information that comes to you through your senses, your knowledge, and your values, you create an inner world based on the outer world you've encountered. This inner world we call the *all-we-know world*. It holds everything we are experiencing now as well as everything we can remember; things we have sensed, things we know, things we believe. This is the world in which we truly "live." Most people think of this as our *mind*.

THE QUALITY WORLD

Out of all the information contained in our mind, we each create a very individual and special place where we store the ideas that fulfill our needs best: our *quality world*. Just as in a photo album, here is where we store the "pictures" of who we want to be; what we want in a friend, parent, partner, child; the "best" food, clothing, houses, holidays; our morals and beliefs. These images are the basis for our choices. They tell us what our needs are, and motivate us to fulfill them by holding up a goal.

Most people store in their quality world the foods that satisfy many of their needs (for me it used to be chocolate). Dieters restrict food intake, often disallowing the foods they value most for long periods of time. Dieters often store a picture of "what my life would be like if I were thinner." Dieters imagine their lives in this "thin" world—perhaps they would be more glamorous, better at sports, wear more beautiful clothes, have more loving mates, be more admired and loved.

These images can be unrealistic, but the main problem with them is that they always occur in the future. Where does that leave you in the present? Dieters get "signals" that their quality world doesn't match the real world every time they look in the mirror.

If when you face the scale or the mirror you see a disturbing gap between what you want in your quality world and what exists in reality, you will be discouraged. If you actually attain the "thin world" and every other need in your life is not also taken care of, you will see a gap as well. Dieters often feel terribly urgent signals when they see these gaps between reality and what they value. The signals can feel like *guilt*, or *discouragement*, or even an *urge to eat*.

What if we had a quality world in which our "ideal self" was healthy, energetic, and happy? What if our weight or size simply didn't matter?

This is hard for most dieters to imagine. It might be easier to imagine what the world would be like if diets didn't work. If there were absolutely no way you could diet and make a difference in your appearance, the world might have to accept a completely different attitude toward body appearance. Beauty would be a matter of function; in cold countries a layer of fat might be considered an advantage; clothing might be designed differently!

The main thing, though, would be that you could live in the pleasant present instead of the future perfect.

Signals

Signals are urgent cues to act. They occur when our real world doesn't match up with our quality world. You get signals when your scale doesn't read the way you want, or your clothes feel tight.

Dieters, when they get negative signals, often criticize themselves, promise to eat less, eat and feel guilty for not keeping their promise, and feel awful at their lack of self control.

There is a reason why our actions are not helpful when we get signals. Dieters have undergone a long, hard training in diet thinking, and this kind of thinking sets up conflicting signals. Our signals from food can be very confusing. For example, we see our favorite food (nicely pictured in our quality world and on the counter in front of us), and we think, "That looks tempting!" Almost simultaneously, we think, "It's too high-calorie!" or "I shouldn't eat it," or "I have no willpower."

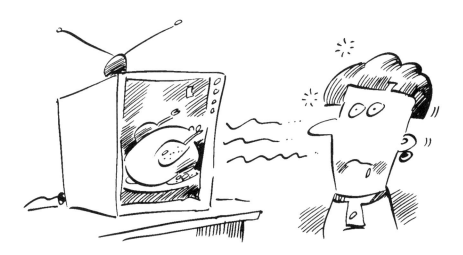

People with eating problems get stronger and more various signals, both positive and negative, about food than natural eaters do. All these conflicting signals can drive us to distraction! It means that food assumes a much more important place in our lives than it needs to.

We Must Act, But We Have Options!

Each of us has a whole range of behaviors we can pull out of our repertoire when we get a signal. Behaviors we have used before, whether they are effective or not, are available to us to use again. Also, we each have the capability of designing completely new behaviors.

Dieters often use eating when they get signals, even signals that may have nothing to do with being hungry. The signal might be:

- It's mealtime and I haven't had lunch yet.
- It tastes good.
- I'm tired/bored/lonely.
- Everyone else is eating.
- I paid for it.
- I'm traveling, I need the energy.
- It's healthy food.
- Mother made it specially for me.
- Better eat the whole meal before dessert.

Say there is a piece of cake on your plate. You have eaten half of it and you feel full. Many dieters would pull out these kinds of behaviors: thought, action, feeling, physiology.

Thought: I shouldn't eat any more. It will make me fat. I don't care. I'll eat it anyway.

Action: Eat it anyway.
Feeling: Guilty. Promising to diet tomorrow.
Physiology: Sluggish.

or

Thought: It's not fair that I can't have it all.
Action: Choose not to eat.
Feeling: Deprived. Angry. (Often translated into "hungry.")
Physiology: Not really hungry, but "emotionally hungry."

Natural eaters rely on hunger signals to help them decide what to eat and when. The hunger signals take the place of conflicting signals. Here is how "natural eaters" combine the elements of thinking, feeling, acting in their eating behaviors:

Thought: My stomach is full. I can't manage any more. That tasted great.
Action: Refrained from eating any more.
Feeling: Satisfied and comfortable.

or

Thought: I am going to feel uncomfortable if I eat this, but I will put up with that for the experience because it's my favorite. I'll just need less to eat later on today.
Action: Eating more.
Feeling: Satisfied, perhaps physically uncomfortable and aware of it, but no guilt or deciding to "diet tomorrow."
Physiology: A little sluggish.

Nectar offers a way to learn a range of new behaviors that include thoughts, feelings, actions and physiological changes, with positive results. When your feelings and thoughts and your body needs are congruent with the actions you choose, you will find it quite rewarding. You will begin to see how good it feels to be in control of your decisions. At the same time, each choice you make will help you think positively, feel satisfied, and take care of your body.

The Thoughts That Lead To Freedom.

These are the six basic beliefs natural eaters have:

- The *all foods are equal* thought: "I am free to consider all foods as equal in their right to nourish me."
- The *selecting* thought: "I am free to give my stomach priority in deciding what it wants."
- The *faith in the future* thought: "My body will look after itself in the future. I am free to trust in the future."

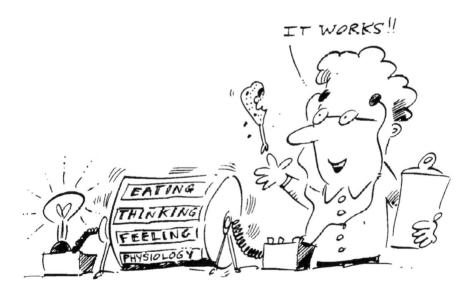

- The *signals* thought: "I am free to listen to the signals my body gives me, and to feel good about what they tell me."
- The *starting* thought: "I can have that any time I want. Do I want it now?"
- The *stopping* thought: "Will my stomach feel better over the next hour if I eat the rest of this? I am free to eat as much as I want."

These are the beliefs that make people into natural eaters. Reading them now you may be thinking, "I don't get it. They sound wrong! And anyway, what do they mean exactly?"

It certainly isn't enough to memorize these statements and repeat them to yourself by rote. You need to believe them. And to believe them, of course, you must have proof. Let's start with the first one.

$\mathcal{C}hapter\ 6$

ALL FOODS ARE EQUAL

I am free to consider all foods equal in their right to nourish me.

Here's a fact that comes as a surprise to most dieters: You are like that little hummingbird on the cover, free to choose whatever you want to eat! You can roam free, settling in one place, then another, taking some of the best of everything, sipping at each, enjoying what you eat, tailoring the amount to what your body needs. Hummingbirds are natural eaters! They eat just enough to satisfy, often sharing the flower's offering of nectar with a bee. In a hummingbird's world, there are many blossoms, of many different species, all competing to attract the bird and the bee by offering the best of what they can prepare. Fields full of flowers have dressed their nectar in beautiful colors and made it attractive in shape and perfume as well as taste.

If you picture yourself like that hummingbird, and the variety of foods available to you like the flowers in that field, you will be making a start towards developing our first thought—that all foods are equal in value. Imagine the whole scene, filled with flowers of all kinds, competing for the attention of the bird. Think of all the foods available to you as well, competing for your attention. You have the freedom to choose.

Freedom

One of the principles of control theory we use in Nectar is that we have the freedom to choose. Freedom is one of our five basic needs. We must exercise freedom, or we will feel frustrated in our lives. This, of course, is one of the reasons diets don't work!

At the moment, conventional dieters' wisdom divides food into "good" and "bad," according to whether it is high in calories, fat, sugar, or cholesterol. Everything tempting is "bad." Part of the reason certain foods become so tempting is that they were prohibited, or severely limited. I can remember when potatoes and bread were limited on diets; they were so temptingly unattainable then! These days, as "recommended" diet foods, they have lost some of their attraction!

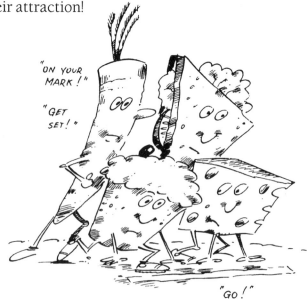

NECTAR THINKING:

All foods are competing on their merits for a place in your stomach.

Like the hummingbird, you are free to choose from among them *all* to satisfy your needs.

Exercise:

Here's a useful exercise to help you picture this and practice it. I call it the Food Olympics. Imagine a race in the Olympic Games for items of food to enter, and the gold medal was a place in your stomach. Suppose, for example, that a carrot, a cupcake, a piece of cheese, and a tuna sandwich are lined up at the starting blocks, ready to compete in a hurdles race. There are six hurdles. The first five are your senses.

The first hurdle is your *sight*—how each of them looks. Is the piece of cake a little ahead at this point? To me, the carrot looks a little hard. The cheese is quite uninteresting to look at; the tuna sandwich seems more interesting, especially in color contrast, so it is probably coming a very close second, if not tying with the cake.

They all approach the next hurdle, your sense of *smell*. The cheese caught up a little here, the sandwich is still going well, the carrot smells fresh. Maybe the cupcake just got a little farther ahead.

Now, your sense of *touch*— the feel of each of them in your

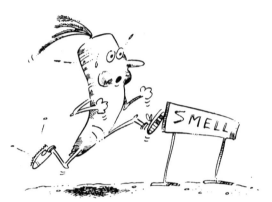

mouth—imagine it! Maybe the carrot is catching up a little? It is harder, perhaps cooler? Does the cheese catch up?

Next, the *taste*. Imagine the taste of each. Every one of us is going to have a particular preference here.

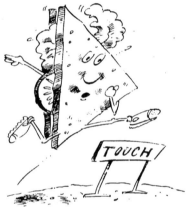

Now the fifth hurdle—*sound*. The carrot just put on a great turn of speed—it sounds really crunchy!

So far, the cupcake has been doing well because for most of us it pleases our senses. Perhaps the tuna sandwich is doing well, too.

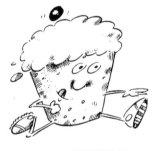

There is a last hurdle, the highest one of all. This last hurdle is how it will *feel* in your stomach.

Once you imagine the cake in your stomach, you need to consider whether it can jump that last

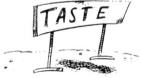

hurdle, and for this, your stomach has to be ready for it! Could be that the amount of fat and sugar doesn't feel right at this point; the cupcake just fell back and the carrot sailed ahead! Or did the tuna sandwich or the cheese feel better?

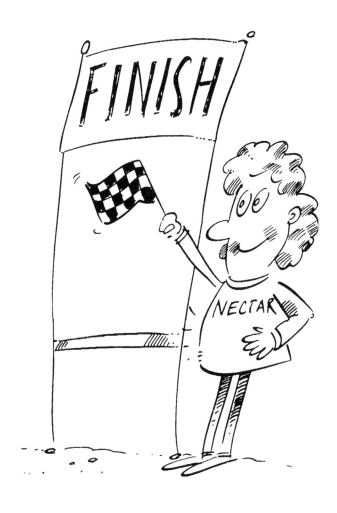

What is important here is not so much *what* you choose on each occasion, but the idea that any food you consider eating needs to start on an equal basis with everything else, and go over that last hurdle.

What used to happen for me, before I completely understood these ideas, was that because the cake was forbidden, it could just go right past that last hurdle without jumping it. Foods that were forbidden had an automatic advantage and could start the race halfway down the track!

If every food has to compete on its merits with every other food for the prize of being given room in your stomach, you will find that your attitude toward selecting the right food becomes quite different.

After all, room in your stomach *is* precious, and worth competing for. It is limited, just the way you used to believe that your access to forbidden food was limited.

Now everything is turned around—it is your stomach that is the prize instead of the food. A good place to try out this idea would be at a smorgasbord or all-you-can-eat food bar, where there is a wide selection of dishes. Go along the display, and imagine that every one of those dishes is competing for a place in your stomach. Would you mindlessly sample each one, not considering whether you liked it or not, getting all the tastes mixed up, just because they were there? Or would you look them all over, think about your own Olympic track, and make a decision about which ones would really win? If you keep remembering that last hurdle, and how it is getting higher every time you take a mouthful because your stomach is getting fuller, you can negotiate a smorgasbord with great pleasure!

NECTAR THINKING:

The only foods that pass my lips are foods that I like.

If you try this just once, you'll know how *great* it feels. From now on, you should make sure that everything that passes your lips is something that you enjoy. If you are not enjoying it, give yourself and your stomach a break— leave it! Nothing terrible will happen.

Always eat what you like first; no more keeping the best till last so that the taste will stay with you longer. As a child you were probably told to eat everything on your plate. You're grown up now—eat the tasty things first and leave what you don't want. Think of food as *serving* you rather than *controlling* you. Live in the pleasant present!

Example:

Janet had been practicing Nectar for a while when she called one day to say, "I've just eaten my first half donut." I said, "What do you mean?" She said, "Well, I was in a cafe with my sister for morning tea. We have both been dieting for years, and our usual 'tipple' is a pot of tea and a rice cake, because it's low-calorie. My sister said, "Are you having ricecakes?" and I said, "No, I'm going to have a donut! I haven't eaten one for so many years and I always want one when I come here.

"She stuck to the rice cake, and with great pleasure I picked up the donut. To my surprise, it was nowhere near the delectable taste I expected and had been yearning for. In fact, I didn't really enjoy it very much, so I left half of it. Next time, I can choose much more freely between the donut and the rice cake, and I have a feeling that the rice cake might just win."

Janet used to go home and console herself with something sweet because she felt deprived. Her total calorie intake would end up higher than if she had eaten just as much as she needed of what she wanted, and felt satisfied. Now that she feels the freedom to choose what will satisfy her at any given time, there's no "aftermath eating." Just natural eating.

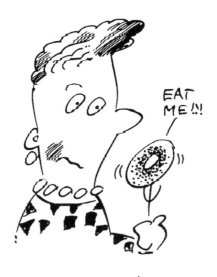

THIS IS WHAT ALL THE FUSS HAS BEEN ABOUT?!!

NECTAR THINKING:

Eat what you like but first think about what you like.

Don't assume donuts are the only food for you; don't assume you hate carrots. Let each food jump the hurdles; then, notice whether or not you're really enjoying it. If you're not, put it down. Don't inflict it on your stomach. And have something else next time. What you are doing is exercising your freedom to eat whatever you want, as well as taking the responsibility (the flip side of freedom) to treat your stomach with the respect it deserves.

As you learn the thoughts that help you to feel good while you do this, your body will begin to take charge of your weight.

Example:

Karen, a former instructor for a well-known weight-reduction plan, told me this after she had been doing Nectar for about eight weeks:

"The thing that is so exciting for me is cheese. I used to boast when I lectured that if you looked in my fridge, it would be empty between the freezer and the crisper— and I was proud that I could keep it that way. Now, it's full of cheese (every kind I like) and I feel so comfortable just having it there that I don't really need to eat it. In fact, often it goes moldy and I throw it away. It's enough to just have it available."

Karen had become a weight-loss instructor so that she would be able to keep herself on a diet, and it worked for her for a long time. She was satisfying her power need by looking good and by knowing that she was helping other people. She kept thin for years. When she gave up the weight-loss instructor's job, the habits she had learned did not sustain her anymore, because she still felt bad about food. Her needs were not balanced because she was restricting her freedom around food, and she still felt controlled by food. She was not exercising her freedom to choose.

Power

Control theory tells us that another of our basic needs is power. This is not just power over people or things, but power to choose and to act. Whenever we make choices about food, we are exercising our need for power and freedom both—as well as feeding our stomachs. We *must* exercise our power in order to live balanced, healthy lives. Natural eaters exercise their power in many ways, not the least of which is by thoughtfully choosing when and what they eat.

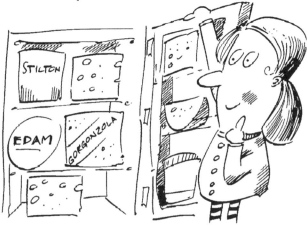

HMM! NOT RIGHT NOW !!!

NECTAR THINKING:

We choose all our behaviors.

You may be starting to realize this about behavior. We choose it! Whenever we behave, we *choose* what we do. Sometimes the behavior doesn't *feel* like a choice, but it is.

Whether we eat a tuna fish sandwich, or six carrots, or a donut or three—we are in charge of deciding. Some of us haven't had much practice deciding what to eat for ourselves in a thoughtful way. But we still make choices. We have that power, and that freedom, too. Other people or circumstances don't decide for us what we will do.

The evidence for this is very clear, once you think about it. Take for instance two children who swim in the surf for the first time. A wave knocks them both over. One screams and rushes out, the other laughs and looks for more. Did the wave itself cause those behaviors? Obviously, the wave was responsible for knocking them over physically, but did it determine how each of them felt? Or was the feeling (for one child fear, for the other enjoyment) a product of their beliefs and thinking?

Now, imagine the difference between me and an answering machine. What happens when the phone rings? If I'm not home, the answering machine picks up after four rings. If I *am* home, I can pick it up, or let the machine do it for me, depending on whether I am busy. I have a choice to make each time it rings. Do I want to answer it or not? It's all up to me, and it depends on what *my* needs are at the time. Am I busy? Am I looking forward to hearing from a friend? Might it be a business call? My need (for freedom, love or power) and what I am thinking and feeling affects my decision. The ringing phone can't make me answer it. I choose to, or not.

NECTAR THINKING:

We act according to what happens inside us.

What we choose to do, and its consequences, are our own responsibility. This means, also, that we can't make anybody else do anything. The only influence we have on other people's behavior is to give them information (in whatever form—sometimes very persuasive, such as a loaded gun) and let them decide what they will do.

Food cannot make us eat it either. We are always choosing whether we eat it or not. It really doesn't have even the persuasive powers of a loaded gun, though sometimes the message we give ourselves feels as strong as that.

Example:

Jonathan had problems with this concept. He said, "But sometimes we have no choice. Yesterday, as my parents

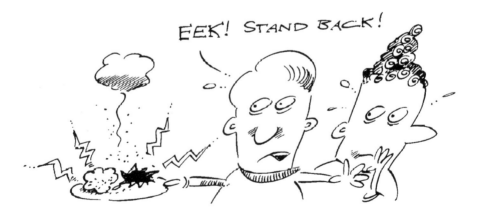

EEK! STAND BACK!

were leaving, we were out in the street as they got into their car. My mother handed me back the baby. I had no choice whether I took her or not. I *had* to take her."

I said, "Yes, you did have a choice. There were a number of things you could have chosen to do. You could have not put your arms out offering to hold the baby, or you could have asked your mother to give her to someone else, or suggested that she take her with her."

Jonathan said, "But none of those things would have been acceptable. The only. . . . Oh, I see what you are saying: my best choice was to take her!" In this case, Jonathan did have a number of choices of action that he had rejected as unacceptable—so unacceptable that he probably didn't even think of them. Many times, a choice does not feel like a choice, but it still is one. Sometimes we choose our behavior without recognizing that we are doing so.

Sometimes our choice of action is limited by circumstances we didn't choose. Hostages or prisoners, for example, suffer certain limits on their freedoms. And we have all seen little children sitting in a stroller, screaming to be let out. But they still have the power and freedom to make certain choices. They don't have a physical choice about where they can go. But they do choose what they think and how they feel. By crying, babies are acting to let their parent know that they don't like whatever is happening. Prisoners exercise their power and freedom needs when they try to escape; they could feel more free and powerful by simply performing mental and physical exercise. They are acting on the world with the best behavior they can come up with at the time to make it the way they want it to be. The behavior may not work, but it is still within their power to choose it.

Example:

Judy's phone rings; she leaves the ironing to answer it (no conflict there!) and her friend tells her something they were going to do together has been canceled. Judy feels disappointed. As she puts down the phone, she thinks, "What do I want to do now? I think I'll have a break." She puts on the pot for some coffee, and thinks, "Maybe just a cookie." She chooses the coffee and cookie, even if she isn't in the least bit hungry, because she will "feel better" after it. This is faulty thinking: the "feel-better" behavior that she is choosing is really only physiological, not emotional. And once the food has gone (sometimes just out of her mouth) the "feel-good" signal disappears and she then starts another behavior of self-criticism because she has eaten something "bad for her." Now she has an even stronger, negative signal, composed of the original bad news *and* the guilt about having eaten the cookie.

She Made Me Do It

Each time, Judy has made a choice of behavior. The choice has related not just to the action, but also to what she believed, what she thought and how she felt. Think about how you explain to yourself things that happen to you. Have you ever said to yourself things like these?

- I shouldn't hurt the hostess's feelings, so I must eat it all.
- My family is expecting me tomorrow, so I have to go.
- My friend made me angry when he insulted me.

If this is how you explain things to yourself, even if you don't say these things out loud, then you are express- ing the belief that other people make you behave. You are using what I call "helpless" language. This doesn't mean that you necessarily change the behavior you choose—it just means that you recognize it as a choice. Turn around those sentences to see that you are really in control:

- I am *choosing* to consider the hostess's feelings, so I am *choosing* to eat it all.
- The family is expecting me tomorrow, so I *choose* to believe that they really want me there, and I *choose* to go.
- I *chose* to feel angry when my friend insulted me.

Doesn't it feel different when you put it that way?

Turning the language around doesn't mean that you should change what you do, or that you shouldn't feel the

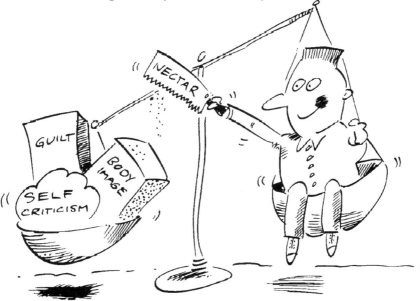

way you choose to feel—you may well be justified in sticking to your choices. But once you recognize your choice, you have a lot more control over what you do. As soon as you say to yourself, for instance, "I am choosing to feel angry." The next thought is often: "How long do I want to choose to feel angry? If it is a choice, is it doing me any good?"

If I want to feel angry, I can keep on doing so. (Aha! Hear the freedom coming in here?) Or, I can decide to do something else. What would be the most effective behavior for getting me what I want? Anyway, what do I really want? You can see how much more control you have over what you do when you recognize the choices you have.

So How Does All This Apply Too Food?

What it helps us to realize is that life is made up of lots and lots of choices—little behaviors which, as they add up, make a huge difference in how we live. The more we are conscious of making satisfying choices, the more balanced our lives will be.

Many choices we make are so habitual that we don't even realize that we are making them. This is what has happened in unnatural eating. If you think back to the way we have become used to filtering information about food, you can see how our choices have become almost automatic, especially our thoughts and feelings.

Start "catching your thoughts." Become more conscious of what you are telling yourself when you are selecting, starting and stopping, in relation to food. Find the "should" thoughts. Change them round to "choose" thoughts.

NECTAR THINKING:

"I can have that any time I like.
Do I want it right now?"

Stop and say this to yourself whenever you are thinking
"I've *got* to have that donut." Think it over. *Then* make
your choice.

Example:

George has a job where he is driving around all day. He
used to eat automatically whatever his wife had packed
for him in the car until it was finished. He ate a lot of
food, but he didn't really enjoy it. He decided to start
choosing his own food and snacks so that they would be
more satisfying. He found that the cookies he chose didn't
disappear the way he thought they would; after he had
munched just a few he felt happy and contented. What
had happened before was that his wife had chosen his
food for him. Once he started making his own conscious
choices of what he would eat, he noticed that his clothes
were getting looser.

Example:

Jenny went to a buffet in Las Vegas where the range of
choice was just amazing. Ordinarily, she would have
taken a little of everything just because it was there and
she could have as much as she wanted. This time, she
made a choice: she surveyed the whole lot, then selected
some seafood and a few other tasty morsels. When she
really tried them, she found that they didn't really taste
as good as they looked, and she left most of the main
meal. Dessert was the same: she took samples of ten

different ones and tasted a little of each, went back for a little more of one she had enjoyed and left the rest. She was surprised that she was disappointed in the buffet overall—the *quality* of the food was important to her, not the *quantity*. Making her choices led to this significant piece of learning.

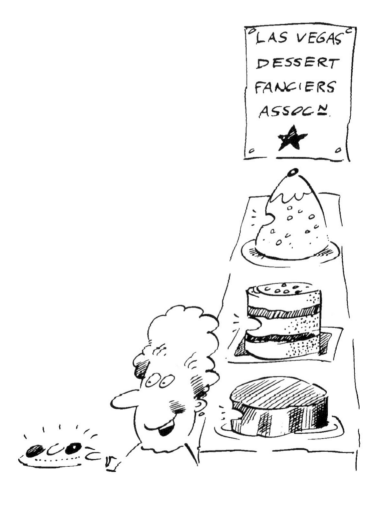

- All foods are equal.
- All foods are competing on their merits for a place in my stomach.
- The Food Olympics Hurdles:
    How does it *look*?
    How does it *smell*?
    What is the *texture*?
    How will it *taste*?
    How will it *sound* when I chew?
- The only foods that pass my lips are foods that I like! I will eat what I like, but first I'll think about what I like, and choose.
- How will that food feel in my stomach?
- Is this the best quality food I can find?
- Which of these foods do I *really* want?
- I choose all my behaviors.
- I act according to what happens inside *me*.
- Food cannot make me eat it. I am in charge of choosing what I eat.

Chapter 7

THE SELECTING THOUGHT

What happens at hurdle number six?

I am free to give my stomach priority in deciding what it wants.

Remember that sixth hurdle in the Food Olympics? Which food made it over the hurdle for you, and how did you decide? If all foods are to compete on an equal footing for a place in your stomach, then we need some way of working out which one wins!

Here are some ideas that will help you negotiate the sixth hurdle. Unstretched, your stomach is about the size of your fist. It helps just now to know how much room the foods are competing for.

Go back to our four competitors, the carrot, the cupcake, the cheese, and the tuna sandwich. Sit quietly, close your eyes, and imagine them, one at a time, sliding down your food passage and into your stomach. Think about how each of them feels to you as it sits there. This is going to be determined to some extent by the condition your stomach is in at the time. The body actually has its own wisdom and will select what it needs, if we really give it a chance.

Animals' bodies have their own wisdom; each variety is programmed to eat just what will suit it. Koala bears, for example, eat only the leaves of certain types of eucalyptus. That is probably one reason why people have not tried to domesticate them. It is simply too difficult to ensure their food supply. How do they know which leaves suit them? It must be that their bodies are programmed to know what will suit their stomachs.

We can identify the same wisdom in all animals. They know whether they are carnivores, herbivores, or omnivores. Humans are omnivores, which gives us the widest selecting capability. What we have done with our natural wisdom is to overlay it with a huge amount of external information, which means that we seldom give our bodies a chance to exercise their own biological knowledge.

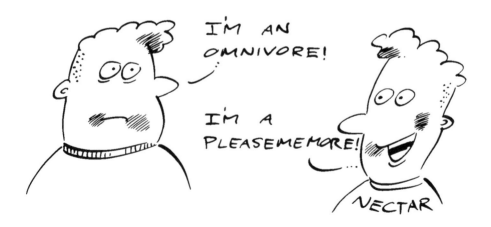

THE THREE FILTERS AND HOW THEY WORK

Information flows through three screens, or filters in order to reach our minds. If these filters are clogged or otherwise not functioning well, they can skew information in such a way that we choose behaviors that are not helpful.

Senses Filter

Think about the senses in relation to food. Some people seem to have a stronger sense of smell and taste than others. For example, people who smoke may find that their senses filter does not operate as well as that of a non-smoker, and therefore they don't receive strong taste-smell signals. Smell is also a sense that evokes memories and emotions connected with them. For me, roasting lamb brings back the Sunday mornings of childhood and family discussions. Our visual sense is important, too, in eating. Many people probably get almost as much pleasure out of looking at a dessert as out of actually eating it, but many times the taste doesn't come up to the promise of the appearance. Just like in the Food Olympics, eating involves all of our senses: sight, touch, taste, smell and even hearing (the difference between squashy and crunchy, for example).

Knowledge Filter

Dieters' knowledge filters are contaminated by all sorts of uncomfortable information, such as the calorie or fat content of so many foods, the images we have absorbed of the "ideal" bodies of fashion models. This information, whether fed to us by advertisements or medical studies, can obscure reality. For example, medical studies frequently contradict each other. What the ads *don't* tell you are facts like these: ten years ago, women who got jobs as models were 3% below the recommended weight for their height. These days, they are 25% below the recommended weight. How unrealistic is the picture we have of an "ideal" body!

Try to imagine living in this world with a knowledge filter that had no information in it about what, when, or how much to eat. It knew nothing of calories, scales, mealtimes, taste, models, clothing, and mirrors. What would you do to survive? Wouldn't your body's welfare be the most important factor in deciding what you put in your mouth?

The only guidelines you could use would be signals from your stomach telling you whether it was hungry or satisfied, and from your whole body telling you how what you ate was affecting your well-being. You would probably be able to judge that by how much energy you had. If you were a hummingbird or a koala bear, you would know exactly what to eat, no worries!

Values Filter

Contained in our values filter are all the beliefs or myths about food, weight, eating, and appearance that we have learned from childhood experiences or discussions with people, school, and the media. Many of these beliefs are the cause of our overeating problems.

Some of the most dangerous myths are old ones such as:

- It is important to clean your plate, because you must not waste food.
- People who are fat have more problems than people who are not.
- You must eat the main course before dessert.
- All sweet things are bad for you.
- To be acceptable, you should look like the people on TV.
- At breakfast,you must eat enough to keep going till lunch time.

As information goes through our values filter, we make it either positive, negative, or neutral. For unnatural eaters, food is valued in an overly positive way. It has become too important. But at the same time, because of all the conflicting information in the knowledge and values filters, food has an overly negative value. Food is both positive and negative at the same time! We view it as enticing but deadly (that chocolate bar) or legal but dull (a stick of celery). Natural eaters put a lower value on food, so that it is pleasant but more neutral. For them, it has none of the agony of conflicting values. They can see all foods as OK.

This is why dieters have such trouble with Hurdle Six. Instead of listening to our body to see what it wants, we let our supercharged value of food—both positive and negative—plow right around the hurdle to avoid those awful conflicts.

Learning To Jump That Last Hurdle

How in the world can an unnatural eater jump that hurdle cleanly? Mostly by focusing on something more important than all those conflicting thoughts: focusing on your *body*. Let's try those Food Olympics again and see how you can use your imagination to master hurdle six.

It's early morning. I know my stomach is empty. The carrot, cupcake, tuna sandwich, and cheese are at it again. First one to reach the hurdle is the cupcake. I imagine it in my mouth first: the icing is a little sweet, and apart from a slightly greasy sensation, the taste is quite good. As it goes on down, it sits there a bit leaden, perhaps a little too much sugar for this time. If it was way ahead in the race through the senses, perhaps just part of it might make it over the hurdle.

What happened to the cheese? Oh, no! It just doesn't get over at all. It feels so heavy, quite uncomfortable. The tuna sandwich now—perhaps part of it might get there. The bread feels quite good, the lettuce feels kind of crisp and crunchy, and the tuna feels OK too, so long as it isn't a huge amount. The carrot? It feels really good: light, crisp, fairly solid, and somehow "nourishing," which I think is my body wisdom speaking (yesterday I gave my body very little vegetable matter, and I think it is asking for some today). What a surprise! As a long-term dieter, carrots have not been my favorite food; they represent the "substitute" food. (Keep carrots in the refrigerator, and eat one when you are hungry). They were "legal, but dull." But putting them through the sixth hurdle, and letting them compete equally with other foods, changes their character completely. The reason for eating them today is so different from my old reasons. When there is no negative information attached to them, they feel (and more importantly, I feel) quite different. There is no "should" attached; I have exercised my freedom instead of my guilt. I might have received a different answer if I had eaten differently yesterday, but that is how it should be; we should be able to select what is "right" in our stomachs, and this process will help us.

When you hit that sixth hurdle, stop and check in with yourself with these questions:

- I can have whatever I want. What will feel right?
- If that piece of food were in my stomach, how would my stomach feel?
- How can I treat my body well?
- What does my body really want?
- How would that food feel in my body right now and for the next hour?

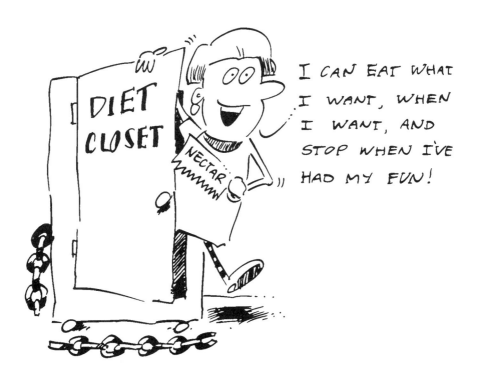

Chapter 8

FAITH IN THE FUTURE

My body will look after itself in the future. I am free to trust in the future.

Here's a surprising bit of information: your body is actually programmed to keep itself at the weight at which it functions best.

Evidence from experiments tell us that when people are asked to put on weight, they can do so. But when the experiment is over they return to their previous weight without effort. The reverse, however, is not true. When we try to lose weight fast, our bodies resist the changes and go into "famine" mode.

The Minnesota Study

In Minnesota, after World War II, a group of men who had no history of weight or eating problems volunteered to participate in a study. They were to lose 25% of their body weight. Following the experiment, they weighed 10% *more* than before they started, and were 40% fatter.

Even more interesting were the behavioral and psychological reactions of these men. They were anxious about food, were overly preoccupied with food thoughts, had food daydreams, talked constantly about food, and had a fascination with cookery and menus. Some ate secretly and guiltily, had difficulty concentrating, and withdrew from people. After the study, many of them continued to have problems with food and eating, and even complained of still being hungry after eating. Does this sound familiar?

It's not a matter of eating less, it's a matter of thinking differently. Why then, you ask me, should I trust in the future? Does this mean that after all my diets my body no longer knows what weight it should be? Am I destined to be forever fat?

The answer to that is no, not if you can learn to think differently. It seems eminently logical that if you eat more to put on weight, then you should just eat less to take off weight, like the Minnesota men tried to do. That is what the world believes, and what has meant years of pain for many of us.

Yet, when we look at the long-term results of restricting our food intake, we see that the outcomes are not what we expected. The Minnesota men did not return to their natural weight, and they ended up with a lot of painful behaviors. There must be another factor that made the difference. This is the secret that can turn around your life in relation to food.

The difference is in what people expect to happen— their view of the future. Natural eaters who are asked to eat more to put on weight "artificially" (as an experiment) do not expect to remain fat. They just know that their bodies will go back to normal when they eat normally again. They do not *try* to get thin. They trust their bodies to return to their natural weight, and their bodies do just that. Their thought patterns about their bodies include the thought "My body will look after itself. I am OK right now."

The Minnesota men who went in the other direction and had a long-term goal to *lose* weight, ended up with a major long-term problem. First, their bodies resisted their attempts to get thinner. At the same time, their thinking and expectations changed. The experiment had planted the new (for them) thought, "I must be thinner, I must eat less than I need." Their bodies were no longer the way they expected them to be. They lost sight of how to eat "normally." The connection in their thoughts between eating and body weight became too strong. They could no longer trust their bodies to return to their natural weight: they had to interfere with their own natural eating habits!

Natural eaters *know* that their bodies will go back to their natural weight. Unnatural eaters try to force their bodies to lose weight, based on the belief that they must get thinner in the future.

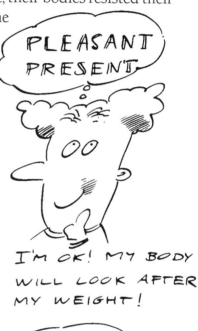

I'M OK! MY BODY WILL LOOK AFTER MY WEIGHT!

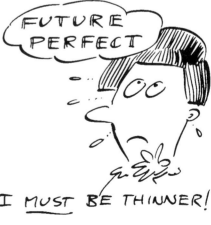

I MUST BE THINNER!

It is not really quick and simple to change the belief that in order to reach the weight we want to be we must limit our eating. But that is what Nectar thinking does. You must trust in the future and enjoy food the way the hummingbird does, eating "enough for now."

How do our quality worlds get stuck in the "future perfect"?

If we go back and look at control theory, we can see what the problem is. As we behave to satisfy our needs, we build up in our heads a large number of "pictures" of what would really suit us best. For example, I am sure that you have in your head a picture of your ideal appearance. Looking good satisfies our needs in all sorts of ways:

- It satisfies our power need by gaining approval or admiring comments from other people.
- It satisfies our love and belonging needs by attracting people we want to have as friends or lovers.
- It satisfies our fun and freedom needs. When we are healthy we can enjoy sports or exercise and feel free to do whatever we want.

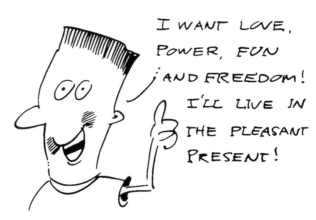

So it is natural to have this "slim" picture in your head as need-satisfying. The problem is that at the same time we have pictures of what foods would be most satisfying to eat. Food also can satisfy most of our needs. The pictures of "ideal body" and "ideal food" conflict!

When we diet, we rigidly hold the "ideal body" picture at the front of our "picture album," and whenever we look at "ideal (or favorite) foods," we push that picture away, telling ourselves how much better we will look in the future by denying ourselves what we really want. This works for a while. The length of time depends on how strong the "body" picture is, and how well we can deny our need for the freedom to eat "ideal" foods.

What happens when we go off the diet is that we gradually let the "food" picture come forward because it is so much more need-satisfying to enjoy our freedom to choose. This also happens when we binge, but in that situation we have the two pictures actively fighting, with the "body" picture producing self-criticism and the "food" picture producing comfort.

Example:

Nora saw her job as a legal secretary as rather dull. She was meeting her need for power mainly by working every minute and producing lots of well-typed pages. Her feeling of importance from other people came from being praised for getting the work done quickly and efficiently, but the work itself she found repetitive and boring. She felt she had very little choice or freedom.

Eventually she decided either to find a way to bring more choices and more responsibility into the present job, or to look for another job where she could have a chance to make more choices within her job description. Having more choices each day would help her to take the stress off her eating patterns and she would not meet her freedom need by eating everything in sight.

The funny thing is, Nora's body actually looked the way she wanted it to look—she was slim and attractive— but she was still focusing on keeping it that way in the future. She needed to let go of the strong connection between her "ideal body" and her eating, and trust that her body would look after its own weight.

Her strategy to work on her needs through her job was a good one, but it would not work long term if she did not also plant in her mind the thought "I am free to trust in the future" in regard to food.

Living In The Pleasant Present

Once you begin to live in the pleasant present instead of the future perfect, life changes. This is because your beliefs and expectations are different. Without "thin body" as a dominant picture in your quality world, your whole view of life changes. Suddenly there are no legal and illegal foods. Thoughts of eating no longer dominate. It is possible to do what a natural eater does:

- Consider your body as a complex system that needs food for fuels instead of being just what you see on the outside.
- Think much more about what each food would do to satisfy your body rather than what damage each food would do to its appearance.

When you live in the pleasant present, you find that you can eat just one chocolate from a box. You find a half-eaten packet of former "binge food" sitting forlornly in the pantry, forgotten. You buy some of your favorite ice cream and throw half of it away because you have had "enough for now." You feel free to go anywhere, eat anything that is around, because you know that food cannot control you.

Maybe, at this stage you think that this is impossible. But why should it be less possible for you than for the natural eaters who *can* do this? They don't have any monopoly on natural thinking, and their bodies really are not made any differently from yours. Dieting has not destroyed any of your natural functions. Your body does still "know" how it was meant to be. If you give it your trust, it will go back to what it was programmed to be.

You may be asking, "But how do I change the way I think? I feel stuck in the future perfect."

The best place to start is with this: Reduce as much as possible the number of times every day that you criticize yourself.

We have been taught that self-criticism is a good way to motivate ourselves. But all it really does is to give us feelings of guilt or anxiety, which we then try to calm down by eating! Wanting to feel good is a much more effective motivation. So what are some of these sources of self-criticism? And how do we get rid of them?

Clean Out Your Closet

The first source of self-criticism for dieters is hanging in your closet. Before Nectar, I had in my closet three kinds of clothes:

- "Hope clothes," left over from when I was thin, or bought in the expectation that I would "fit into them later."
- "Safety nets" (and often that is what they looked like) for when I got fatter again.
- The things that actually fit me at the time.

The closet was always pretty crowded! Did it help me to see all those clothes that wouldn't fit? About as much as beating myself over the head with a broom. Not only that, there were so many clothes crammed in there that I didn't really know what I *did* have that would fit.

So unless you really *like* feeling bad and beating yourself up, I suggest that you go carefully through your clothing and keep in the closet only the clothes that you like and feel good in. So, it looks pretty empty—the clothes will be less crushed, and getting dressed will be lots easier. Some people actually bundle up the hope clothes and give them to charity. If this is too drastic a step, put them away where you don't have to look at them. As you find the present clothes getting too big, you can go look for others, but it won't happen for some time. This process is not about losing weight fast. I am asking you to settle for the body you have *now*, because now is when you are living. Make it the pleasant present!

Once you have taken out all the hope clothes, if you are not satisfied with what is left, go out and buy something you feel really good in. Pick something in bright, cheerful colors that suit your complexion—something that feels good when it goes on. Dress optimistically! Wear it often. If you dress to feel good, you will look good.

Don't look at sizes. Many people see "the next size up" as a terrible barrier. Hold the garment up to yourself and make a judgment as to whether it will fit. Garment manufacturers are really not all that accurate about sizes, and your well-being is far more important than a size label. Cut out the size labels when you get home—big or small!

Example:

Once, in a store, I remember having a choice between two outfits: one was a size 16, the other was a size 20. The smaller-size one was almost one hundred dollars more than the bigger-size one. I tried them both on three times. I actually looked thinner in the larger-size suit because of its lines. The other one with the smaller-size label looked pretty, but overall, I really didn't look as good in it.

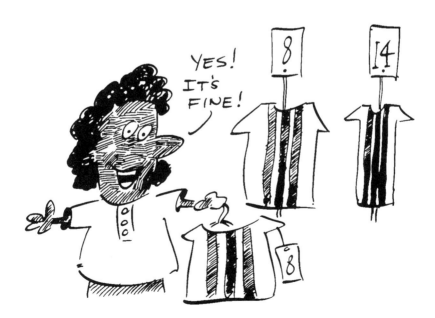

I suddenly realized that the things that *should* be in consideration were how each outfit looked, how I felt in it, and how much it cost. The only thing holding up my decision was a little piece of material labeled "20." Who would ever know about this unless I told them? Did I have to keep that little piece of material in the suit when I got it home? Here I was, considering paying an extra hundred dollars for something I didn't look as good in, just because of a size label! I bought the size 20 and it looked great.

Can you see some new thinking coming in here?

NECTAR THINKING:

If this is the way I am, I'll make the best job I can of looking good.

It's OK to be the way I am. If I am dressed in clothes that look and feel good, being around me will be a pleasant experience for other people because I'll be more cheerful.

Example:

Sarina followed the idea of dressing to please herself; she made herself a new outfit, felt wonderful and went on the train to the city to enjoy herself. In her split skirt she got admiring glances, and thought, "That's pretty good for a dame who's pushing fifty!"

It took me about two years to be so secure in my belief that my new body was permanent that I could also get rid of the "safety nets." I no longer feared that I would need them. So keep the "safety nets," if you must, until you have really internalized your new beliefs.

Dump The Scale

Another source of criticism is the scales. Why should you allow a mechanical device to dominate your life? Go talk to natural eaters, and ask them how often they weigh themselves. I guarantee you'll discover that they weigh themselves rarely or never. They just don't expect their weight to change. Some of us seem to believe that, if we don't weigh ourselves, we will disappear. Let me assure you, that you will still be there—but that little voice that makes you feel bad about your weight may fade away!

Example:

Elizabeth could not face the idea of not weighing herself. She was absolutely certain that if she didn't know how much she weighed, she would probably die. One of the tasks she had to do in the Nectar course was to interview someone who was a natural eater—a person who could truthfully say she didn't have any problems with her weight. She found such a person in the instructor of her aerobics group.

One of the questions she had to ask in the interview was "How often do you weigh yourself?" Elizabeth came back flabbergasted. "She *never* weighs herself! I couldn't believe it!" she said. "She doesn't worry about how much she eats or putting on weight, because she knows she will be the same all the time! That's how I would like to be!" Elizabeth found it very hard to give up her scales, so some of her friends went around one day to visit and removed them from her bathroom. When she found that she continued to exist without the evidence of her scales, she let go of weighing herself, and gradually she lost weight.

People ask me how much weight I have lost, and I have to tell them I don't know. I promise to weigh myself in June—I just don't tell them *which* June. It just is no longer of any importance.

All that happens when you get on the scales is that you give yourself an opportunity to criticize yourself. We

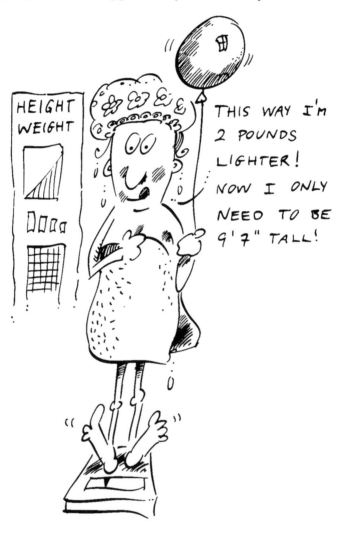

know all the tricks: standing on your toes or your heels, taking off any clothing that might weigh too much. And of course, you *never* eat dinner before you weigh in! The problem is, this strategy only really works once! We try to delude ourselves so that we can feel better about how much we weigh. It's better not to know!

If you weigh more than yesterday, you feel bad and guilty and make a resolution to "be good." Frequently, this lasts only a couple of hours, then we begin eating again and feeling guilty. (Do you recognize the pattern?) Or if we happen to be lighter, we congratulate ourselves and are a little more lenient with ourselves. This means we are still criticizing ourselves for the way we were yesterday and continuing to worry about what we might weigh tomorrow. What an awful way to live life!

If you want to become a natural eater, put away, give away or throw away the scales. They really don't help you to feel good about yourself, and they are an unnecessary source of criticism. If you consider weighing yourself, think, "What the scales tell me doesn't matter. I am letting my body look after my weight." When you started dieting, you had only a 5% chance of success. Getting fat again, or not finishing the diet, is no reason to believe that you have problems beyond those of the majority of people. Dieting is an inefficient behavior that sets up the conditions for failure.

Faith In The Future

My body will look after itself in the future. I am free to trust in the future.

Diets don't work—our bodies resist, and our minds do, too.

I can trust my body to return to its natural weight.

I can live in the pleasant present and forget the future perfect.

Changing how I *think* is the most powerful tool I have in becoming a natural eater.

I will clean out my closet.

I will throw out my scales!

Chapter 9

THE SIGNALS

I am free to listen to my body's signals, and feel good about what they tell me.

Our bodies and minds are constantly giving us signals that are the triggers for choices of behaviors that will fulfill our needs. Some signals we feel in our bodies, others we feel in our minds. Here's a body signal I'm sure you will recognize: the one that says it's time to go to the bathroom. We need this signal to survive—it helps us regulate our body. A clear physical signal such as this, gradually becomes more and more urgent if we ignore it. We might be in an important meeting where our power need is uppermost, or we might be comforting a friend or child and not want to leave. So we feel our body signaling, but we might choose to ignore a physical signal in favor of a stronger psychological signal.

   Mothers and fathers know that the process of training a little child to use the bathroom involves helping the child pay attention to a physical signal, then helping him respond to that signal in a way that satisfies his needs. Eventually, he learns to keep his clothing dry and clean and to act in a way that is acceptable to the standards of the society he lives in. The child learns to obey both physical and psychological signals to complete the process, meeting his physical needs as well as his need for love and acceptance, personal power, and freedom.

Many young children also need help recognizing their hunger signals. We can tell from their behavior that there is something wrong. Maybe they are cranky or report that they feel "sick," and we figure out that they haven't eaten for a considerable time. One mother told me of the terrible drive home she used to have with her preschooler from play group, until she worked out that if she brought a sandwich with her for him to have *before* they got into the car, all was peaceful. Gradually, young children learn to distinguish the different physical signals and to know psychologically what each of them means and how to satisfy them.

When we were children, our signals of feeling hungry or full were quite recognizable, and probably we obeyed them most of the time. Although for many of us, the training we got in how we "should" behave towards food meant that we created many psychological signals that led us to eat for lots of different reasons.

The Two Signals That Tell Natural Eaters To Eat

When you think about it, there are really only two signals that should mean anything in deciding about whether to eat something:

- A physical signal from the stomach.
- A psychological signal that says that there is an opportunity to enjoy the food.

What are some of the other signals we get, though?

- I was good all last week—now I have to have this brownie!
- I feel miserable—maybe if I ate something?
- I'd better eat a balanced dinner—even though I'm not really hungry.
- I hate to leave that on the plate—it looks so good.
- That contains a lot of sugar and fat.
- Mom wants me to show I care by eating this.

All these other signals, and our consequent agonizing, are just "static." We call them extraneous signals. We don't *need* them to help us make choices about our food needs. All we need is a stomach signal, or an "I would enjoy that" signal.

What if we are only getting one of these two essential signals? I would enjoy the taste of that! In this case we just need to ask ourselves how much enjoyment we can settle for without getting a physical "full" signal.

With the "I'm hungry" signal, you just decide what would fulfill your hunger (the Food Olympics) and how much you need to be satisfied.

If we really paid attention to *just these two signals*, it would simplify matters considerably. All the extraneous signals would become unimportant—and we could eliminate many of the restrictions we place on what we eat.

NECTAR THINKING:

I can move towards becoming a natural eater.

When I can key my eating to the physical signals of hunger and satisfaction, I will feel free and satisfied.

The Fear-of-Hunger Signal

Unnatural eaters often have an unnatural fear of the hunger signal. Imagine that attached to your stomach there is a barometer, which measures the pressure inside. Unnatural eaters have taught themselves to be afraid of getting hungry. The "low pressure" of hungry is a lot more to be avoided than the "high pressure" of too full. They forget to be concerned about how uncomfortable it feels to eat more than your stomach wants, and how long it can take for the discomfort to go away.

Actually, we should really be afraid to let the needle swing over to "too full." It is much more to be feared than low-pressure hunger. It is much simpler and more pleasant to deal with a hunger signal—you treat it as a chance to enjoy yourself, and eat something. A "too full" signal is much harder to deal with—you can only wait, feeling uncomfortable, for the stomach to process the food (or get rid of the food by vomiting, which is definitely not a desirable way to go!).

Natural eaters know this end of the scale is much more uncomfortable than the hungry end. They take note of the signals their stomachs give as they eat. As

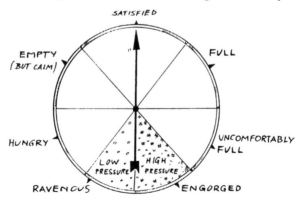

their needle swings to "satisfied," they stop putting more food into their stomachs. No regrets (psychological signals) about having to leave food, no extraneous signals that prompt them to eat more than they need, just simple responses to the needs of their body.

What's Wrong With Being Too Full?

As dieters, we have allowed ourselves to fear hunger signals far more than full signals, because we just know that we will feel bad if we get hungry. We remember that weak-at-the-knees feeling from dieting. This feeling is not related so much to hunger as to another physiologi-

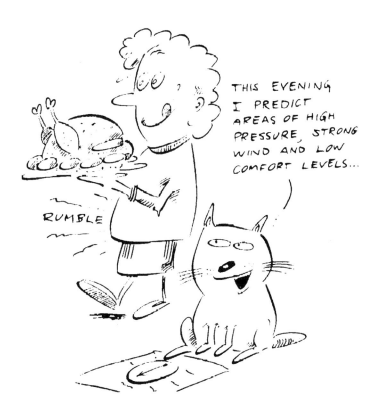

cal change. When you starve your body, it has to get its energy from somewhere, and it takes glycogen first from where it is stored in available form—in your muscles. You won't feel this kind of signal as a natural eater, because you have no reason to starve yourself. You can eat when you need to. We don't think about "too full" signals in the same way, but really they are more to be feared than hunger signals. Most of us reading this are not really living in a situation of true famine. When we get a hunger signal it is usually possible to do something about it right away or in the near future, and have a good experience calming it down.

Fear of hunger used to be logical and sensible, and it comes from our heritage. Parents and grandparents who went through wartime and the Depression had the fear of not knowing where the next meal was coming from, and taught us to make sure we would never let ourselves get hungry. These days, most of us who diet do not suffer a lack of good food. If we're still hanging on to those starvation fears, we need to change our beliefs.

With an overfull stomach, the unpleasant feeling remains for a long time. Quite apart from the obvious physical signal of discomfort, overloading your stomach with food leads to other negative outcomes. Your body will not operate efficiently, and your digestive organs will be put under unnecessary strain.

Unnatural eaters are super-sensitive to the hungry signal, but when it comes to "too full," our brains and our stomachs no longer communicate with each other. The poor old stomach may still be sending along its "full" signals, but the brain is no longer listening! We have trained our brain to do this by—surprise!—dieting. After many experiences of getting the signals from the stomach and ignoring them during dieting, the brain just cuts off the communication channel.

Those signals, and that channel, are still there. It takes time and effort to reopen those channels of communication, but it is quite possible. You have already learned some things about opening those channels in the chapter on selecting. You will learn more in chapters coming up on starting and stopping. First, let's look at those extraneous signals again.

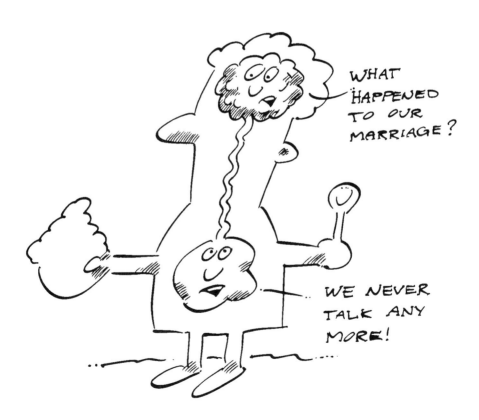

Identify the Two Signals and Ignore the Rest

How can we distinguish between a genuine signal from the stomach and one that comes from our psychological needs? Actually, this is easier than you might think; the first thing to do is to relax about it, to let go of the fear of hunger signals.

Begin to check in with your stomach every time you feel a signal that you interpret as "eat." As you practice, those signals will become easier to interpret. As you focus on your eating signals, it will become clear to you that extraneous signals often relate to other needs—for fun, power, or freedom, for example.

Example:

Jonathan, one of the "experienced dieters" in our first experimental group, had a strong picture of himself having fun in his quality world. For him, fun meant playing table tennis. He hadn't played for a long time, because he felt guilty about going out and leaving his wife to look after their two young children after she'd been home with them all day. So he stayed home, ate everything she prepared—including anything left over that she or the children didn't want, which is a way that many dieters learn to control guilt—and satisfied his fun need to some extent by enjoying the taste of the food.

The group suggested that he go home and strike a bargain with his wife: He would ask her to select a time in the week when she would like a break from the children. He would care for them and she could go out and have fun. In return, she would give him a special time each week when he could play table tennis. She loved the idea. She chose Saturday morning, and he chose Tuesday evening.

As he also learned and practiced more assertive behaviors toward food, he began to match his pictures of himself and feel more in balance in his life. When we asked him at the end of the program what was the turning point for him, he said that it was working on his fun need and realizing that he needed to have fun.

Jonathan had become more conscious of his psychological signals. Once he started listening to the signal he was getting that said, "Have more fun," he changed what he was doing in his life. He stopped listening to the extraneous "eat to please your wife" and "don't waste food"

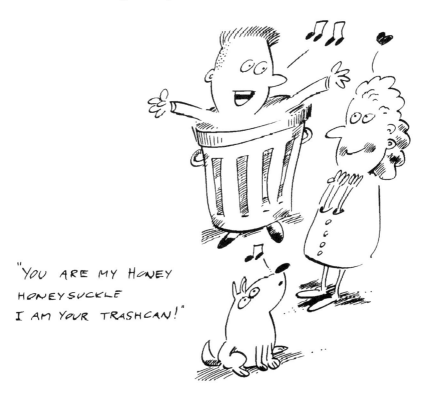

signals and replaced them with "fun for both of us" and "fun for me" signals that he could satisfy by the new arrangements.

Eating And Guilt

One important thing that I noticed about Jonathan's story was that he ate because of a guilt signal. Many of us have developed a strong connection between eating and guilt.

Do you remember the "starving children?" My mother's were in China and their whereabouts seems to depend on the age you were when a famine occurred. The message I got was that I should feel guilty about having a plate of food in front of me that I wasn't eating, because the starving children would be glad to have it. It's the next part of the message that mattered. If you eat it all, you need not feel guilty. You will not be wasting food. This usually wasn't said, but it's the part that we retain long after the starving-children argument is forgotten.

What happens is that we end up with a subtle link between eating and guilt. There are a lot of other ways in which we give ourselves guilt signals:

- Your relatives will be hurt if you don't eat what they have prepared.
- You "should" eat the main course before dessert.
- You "should" eat only healthy food.
- You "shouldn't" eat food that is (you name it!) high in calories, high in fat, high in sugar, produced by underpaid workers—the list is long.

Somehow, in a thousand ways, we associate eating with getting rid of guilt signals. When I examine my binges, that link becomes quite clear. When I felt like eating something "wrong" and ate it, I would feel guilty, and would eat again to get rid of the guilt signal. Many times I would deliberately "shut down" my thinking because it felt too bad. And if there were something I was feeling guilty about beforehand, this would often be the trigger for the binge.

Now that I am aware of it, when I get the old urge to binge (which still happens now and then), I look for what I am feeling guilty about. Usually it is some kind of self-criticism attached to the word "should."

Cutting Through The Guilt

Here is a process you can use to rechannel your thoughts and reduce those guilt signals so that they do not trigger eating. Whenever you feel your "shoulds" raising their ugly heads, check in with yourself by asking the following questions based on a list developed by Diane Gossen, of Chelsom Consultants.

IF I EAT EVERY BIT, I'LL BE GOOD !!

NECTAR THINKING:

We are always doing the best we can.

- Am I being a good friend to myself? If I were my best friend, what would I be telling myself?
- It's not self-indulgence that is making me fat, it's telling myself a "should"!
- Am I free to choose differently next time?

NECTAR THINKING:

All behavior has a purpose.

- I did this for a reason. What do I really want?
- Could I have done something worse? Or, could I have done less, and not addressed the problem at all?
- What worse alternative did I avoid by doing this?
- Though it didn't work out the way I wanted, I was trying to accomplish something; what was it?
- Is there a way to accomplish it more effectively?

NECTAR THINKING:

We are always acting for reasons inside ourselves.

- What value or belief was I protecting by doing what I did?
- Would it be better if I didn't have that value or belief?
- What do I believe about the person I want to be?

Another Way To Check In

When you experience confusing signals about food, try these check-in questions:

- Just what is the *real* signal here?
- Is it physical or psychological?
- What is actually the need behind it?
- Can I work out a way to make the present more truly need-satisfying?
- If I were the person I want to be, what would the signal really mean to me? What could I do to satisfy it best?
- If I choose to eat to satisfy a psychological signal, what would be the tastiest and most need-satisfying thing I could eat? How much of it would leave my stomach feeling comfortable?
- If I wait until I feel hungry will I have a great experience?

Chapter 10

THE STARTING THOUGHT

I can have that any time I want. Do I want it now?

In this chapter, we will teach you how to create a hunger signal, feed it immediately with a small amount of food, feel the signal go away, and see how long it takes to come back.

But, if you are an unnatural eater, you are afraid of getting hungry! You probably remember at some stage of a diet that your legs felt like they were made of jelly. It won't be like that this time because you will eat as soon as you first feel a hunger signal. You had to starve yourself for some time to have that weak feeling.

Hunger signals are the body's way of informing the brain that it's time to renew the available energy. So that is what we are going to do—give the body what it wants! Once your stomach learns that whenever it gives a signal it will be fed, your body and brain will be communicating like those of a natural eater. Your body can take over its function of deciding when it needs to be fed. Communication is a great way to go. Answering a hunger signal becomes quite easy, even fun, once you become accustomed to it again.

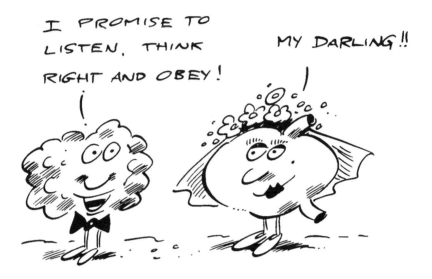

Feeling The Hunger Signal

Have you forgotten what a hunger signal feels like? It's different from empty, when there is no signal, and it comes from your stomach, not the back of the mouth, which can often mean thirst. Mouth-watering is definitely not a hunger signal! It is not easy to predict when a signal will arrive. When you first start waiting for it, the wait can seem endless! Or the signal may come only an hour or so after eating, especially if you haven't eaten much. Morning is probably the best time to do this experiment, because at least you know your stomach is empty.

Example:

The first time I did this, I waited quite a long time. It was after midday and I was driving home after attending one of our experimental Nectar sessions. I hadn't eaten since the night before, and was beginning to despair. Then I felt a signal. At last! I stopped and bought some Thai takeout, and as I got back into the car, a stronger signal arrived. What to do? Wait ten minutes while I drove home? No!

I had a spoon in the car, so I opened a carton and had one spoonful of the gravy. I can still remember the experience after two years. The wonderful taste combined with the magic feeling of the hunger signal easing away at the same time. I didn't know what I had been missing! I timed the return of the signal. It took, believe it or not, half an hour before I got hungry again, and I ate the rest of the food. It amazed me that one spoonful of gravy could have such an effect so fast, and last for so long.

Example:

Julie reported a similar experience. She had the chance to go away to a holiday cottage for a week, and decided to do the hunger-signal experiment. She stopped all the clocks so that she wouldn't be worrying about eating according to the time, and bought all the delicacies that she liked—small amounts of wonderful deli foods. She waited until her body gave a signal, then she ate. It was delightful! Eating exactly what your stomach wants and your mouth enjoys when truly hungry is one of the most delightful experiences you can have. As one of our radio announcers says, it's the best fun you can have standing up!

You should learn three things from this experiment:

- You can actually feel a hunger signal and get a pleasant experience from it.
- The signal goes away fast. There is a myth around that it takes twenty minutes to stop feeling hungry. I find that it's instantaneous. It's the "full" signal that seems less dependable.
- A small amount of food can stop the signal for some time. A very small amount lasts much longer than you would expect.

Example:

Jenny and I were on a country trip in my car. I always carry small amounts of food in my handbag and in the car so that if a signal arrives I can feed it straight away. At exactly the same moment we both said, "I'm hungry!" I searched the car and my bag. All I could come up with was a half a cracker. So, I carefully broke it in half. I felt a bit like a starving sailor in a shipwrecked boat! We ate

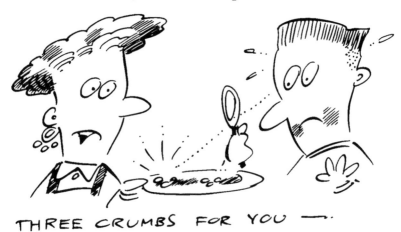

THREE CRUMBS FOR YOU —.
THREE FOR ME !!

our respective quarter crackers; 45 minutes later when we sat down to lunch, neither of us had had another hunger signal.

Tip:

Don't put off starting this experiment with all the excuses that I know you are thinking of: I have to go to work; it will look funny; I have no time; I might lose my energy; I have to have breakfast. . . . Just try it once. It's much more enjoyable than you expect. As I write this, it is 6:00 A.M.; I have been working since 5:00 A.M. I don't expect to get hungry until around 8:30 to 9:00 A.M. at the earliest. By then I will be on my way to a meeting, and I will have something with me. Today it is likely to be half a banana, because that is something I think my stomach would enjoy, but I'll wait till closer to the time and decide. There's always food in my purse, or in the car. Some days, if I'm at home, it might want cereal, or part of a croissant. Remember the Food Olympics, and work on what would feel best.

Example:

Sandra was really worried about how she could eat as soon as she was hungry at work. She was surrounded by other women who, she thought, watched her every move and all the food. There was a custom at lunch time of eating non-fattening foods, because they were all watching their weight. She thought it would be impossible to eat at "out of normal" times, and they would think she was a glutton. She was prepared for the worst! She took the risk, and it turned out that no one even noticed.

I suggest that you try this experiment once, then sit down and think about it so that you see whether your thoughts are the same as I have had. The starting thoughts that you need to make a habit of using are:

- I can have that any time I like. Do I want it now? Is my stomach hungry?
- If I wait until I'm hungry, I can have an extra-special experience.
- Am I hungry or thirsty?

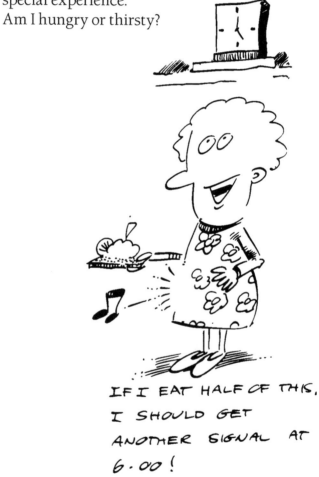

IF I EAT HALF OF THIS,
I SHOULD GET
ANOTHER SIGNAL AT
6.00!

Talking To Your Stomach

I read an article many years ago called "I am Joe's Stomach." It was an account of the chemical processes the stomach used to deal with a ham sandwich. I tried to imagine what my stomach would tell me if it could think and talk. This is how my stomach talked to me:

"I am your stomach, the manager of a factory that has the responsibility for keeping the whole of your body, including your brain, functioning as well as possible. Unless I get raw materials for my factory, I can't do my job. I have no control over what raw materials I get, how many I get or when they arrive, so I have to be very flexible in the way I operate. Ideally, my supplies would arrive so that I could process them without being overloaded. Although I have the capacity to expand my storage space, it is difficult to do the processing efficiently when there is an oversupply of materials. I can send you a signal when I am empty, and increase the strength of the message if you don't hear me the first time.

"The size of my storage capacity is about the size of your fist—that's a good working volume for supplies. If you send me more than a fist's worth, I will send you a signal to say that I really don't need any more supplies right now. I'm sure you can remember the time you sent me a large mass of apple pie with ice cream while I was still working on 'dinner.' It was quite difficult to manage so much at once, because my supply of chemicals was not sufficient to break it all down quickly enough. In fact, I think I sent some back to you on one occasion! I certainly told you that the fat content was very difficult indeed to deal with. My subcontractor, the gall bladder, just could not meet the demand.

"The quality of the supplies is also something you might consider. Certainly, too much grease makes life difficult down here. The best scenario for me would be one where you waited for me to signal you that I need some supplies, and sent me just enough to work on so that I could do it easily.

"What I could do in return would be to keep the level of blood sugars steady so that, your body would feel more energetic and healthy. It would also help if your brain took note of things like whether the raw materials

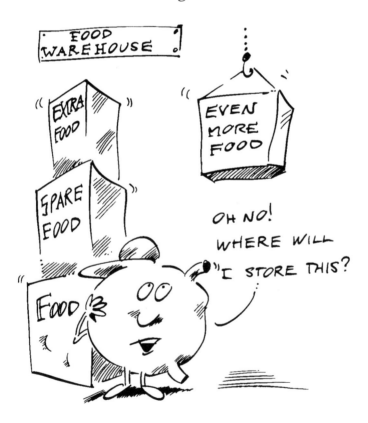

you sent have been the most effective in making your body feel really good, not just right away but an hour or two later as well. If you would pause when you are about to send me some supplies and think about how I might feel about getting them and what I would do with them, I would be happy to let you know whether they would really suit me! If we could just talk more I can promise you some euphoric experiences!"

A woman of many words, my stomach! She seems to know what she's doing. Maybe she could really help! So, what can you do to make your stomach happier? You could start really listening to the signals your body gives you. They have gotten lost in the morass of all the reasons why unnatural eaters eat. But our stomachs are still sending them. It's just that our brains have learned to ignore them. Our dieting taught us to ignore them. We had to stay hungry till it was time to eat. And when we went off our diets we made sure that we didn't ever get hungry!

Many of us are afraid of getting hungry, especially if we have done a lot of dieting. But, as my stomach says, nothing is more enjoyable than eating exactly what you want when your stomach is ready for it. And the hungry signal is much easier and more pleasant to do something about than the overfull signal. Following the hungry signal is logical—and it works.

Illogical Eating

Much of our eating is illogical. For example, whenever I had a long way to travel, I would eat more before I left. This might have been smart if I were going somewhere where there was no food, such as into the desert. But I was

going to places where there would be either coffee breaks
or shops. I would end up eating ahead before I left so that
I wouldn't be hungry, then I would go ahead and have
something else anyway during the morning.

What I do now is to wait until I am actually hungry
before I eat in the mornings. The time of arrival of my
stomach's signal depends on what I have supplied it with
the night before. If I always have something to eat available, I truly have nothing to fear.

Trust Your Stomach

Hunger signals are good. Instead of fearing hunger, understand it as a natural signal that works in our favor.
Being hungry means that we can enjoy eating in two
ways: through our taste buds, and by our stomach's feeling satisfied. Trust that there will always be something
around to eat when our body comes up with its signal.

Tip:

Go grocery shopping for your car, desk, purse and your
briefcase. Keep snacks available wherever you are.

Some of the things you might choose from are
nibble mixes, nuts, crackers, cookies, fruit, juice, dry
cereal, carrots, jerky. I change what I keep in these spots.
At the moment there is a cookie in the car, crackers in a
small container in my purse, special chocolates (the same
brand that got me thinking) in my bedside drawer. I am
always surrounded by food, so that I can afford to eat
sparingly, giving my stomach enough to satisfy it in the
present and for no more than the next hour or so. The
result is many enjoyable eating experiences every day.
Food actually tastes better, not only because my stomach

likes it but also because the act of eating is no longer accompanied by all the furious haste and negative feelings that used to go along with it. Instead, I feel really good about what I eat.

Your Stomach Will Look After Your Body

If you give control of eating over to your stomach, then it will gradually use up all the extra stored energy (fat!) from around your body. It won't happen fast, but because it is slow it will also give you time to make your new natural eating behaviors permanent. And if you happen to overeat now and then, it's no big deal. Your stomach will gradually deal with the extra supplies, probably by not getting hungry as often, or for as much.

Let Go And Let Your Stomach Take Over

You are probably used to your mind keeping control of your weight (the dieter's method), but your stomach already knows how to do that. It tells you what, when and how much to eat. Take care of its needs, listen to its signals, and it will take care of all the rest.

You can relax and let things happen naturally. There is no need to worry about what food might be available, because you are free to eat whatever is there. All you have to do is to work out how much your stomach needs of it. Food is just a pleasant part of your life, there to be thoroughly enjoyed in its place. You are entering the pleasant present!

More Exercises To Try

- You stop for gas as you go shopping or to work. Usually, you would buy a snack as you paid for the gas. Instead, think: "I've got something in the car if I get hungry. Do I really need to buy anything right now?"

- Tonight you are at dinner. Notice whether you are really hungry. You're not? You say you nibbled as you cooked? Consider this: You don't have to eat now. Your stomach doesn't need it! You can put it aside and eat later.

Starting Thoughts

- "I can have that anytime I want. Do I want it now?"
- "I've got something really good at home. Would my stomach feel better if I ate now, or later?"

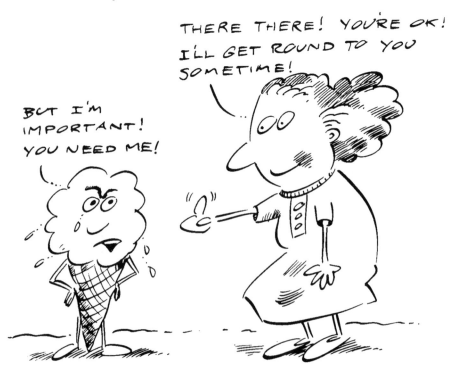

Chapter 11

THE STOPPING THOUGHT

Will my stomach feel better if I eat the rest of this?

Learning to recognize when you have had enough to eat, and to feel good about stopping eating is probably the most important thing you can learn and continue for the rest of your life! Unlikely as it may sound, it is *stopping* that gives you the most freedom. No matter what you want to eat, and even whether you wait until you are hungry or not, if you know how to stop, you will never need to put on weight again.

Stopping is not quite as easy to learn as selecting and starting. This is because the full signal, for us dieters, seems less reliable than the hunger signal. We have learned to ignore it very well! Even natural eaters can't always rely on getting a full signal as soon as they have eaten just enough to make their stomach comfortable.

What often happens is that we finish everything, then a little later we get the signal. But instead of a full signal, it's an overfull signal. Then we feel uncomfortable, and say "I've eaten too much!" The main reason why we stop eating is that all the food is gone! This really has nothing to do with the state of our stomachs.

There is some research that says that the full signal takes about twenty minutes to arrive after the stomach actually fills. I don't know about you, but I know that I can get through an enormous amount of food in twenty minutes. Not only that, but I can ignore *any* signal if I really want to eat the food. So, your thinking process becomes even more important in learning both when to stop and how to feel good about stopping.

How To Stop

Concentrate on getting full instead of worrying about getting fat. Put the emphasis on your stomach and how much it can cope with.

Ask yourself:

· How can I make my stomach comfortable?
· How much does it need to feel good for the next hour?

Think Ahead To Full

You can't really wait for the full signal to arrive. It might come too late. For many of us, after our stomachs signal full, the signal keeps getting stronger, even if we don't eat any more, until we feel bloated and uncomfortable. Rather than sit with a clock and wait for twenty minutes, we need to use other cues (such as looking at the amount of what we are eating) to let us know when to stop. The goal is to draw our eating to a healthy and comfortable close—as if drawing the curtain on a good play.

Enjoy The Performance And Applaud At The End

By the end of a meal you have enjoyed the taste, the eating experience, the variety, and, like at a good play, you feel regret combined with satisfaction as it comes to a close. You might want an encore, but eventually the play ends and you go away satisfied. That's how to end a good meal—satisfied.

Ask yourself the stopping questions:

- Is the rest of the food going to taste better, or just the same?
- Will my stomach feel any better over the next hour or so if I eat the rest?

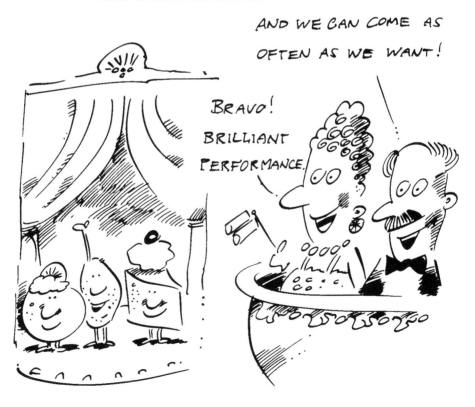

Example:

Recently, I visited an ice cream parlor. Someone had told me about a chocolate brownie ice cream with hot fudge sauce. It sounded decadent and delicious to an old ex-dieter like me. I had no trouble getting over the hurdles in that Food Olympics! At the time I reached the parlor, I wasn't actually hungry, although I hadn't eaten for a while. I ordered this magnificent concoction, in a waffle cone, and sat down to eat it. It really did taste very rich and wonderful—perhaps a little too sweet at the taste hurdle. I ate about six mouthfuls, then asked myself, "Is the rest of it going to taste *better*, or just the same?"

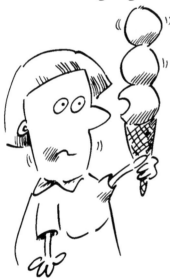

IS THE REST GOING TO TASTE BETTER, OR JUST THE SAME?

The answer, of course, was "just the same." I could prolong the taste another couple of minutes, that's all. I would remember the taste anyway after just a few bites. It would linger on my tongue, and in my memory, even if I stopped now.

So then I thought about my stomach "Will my stomach feel any better over the next hour or so if I eat the rest?"

The answer was, of course, "No." In fact, it would probably feel worse. So I said to myself, "This has been a great experience. I must repeat it sometime." I threw the rest of the cone into a garbage bin and walked out feeling just the way I do after a good play, content and full of pleasure, and with the sweet tang of chocolate on my tongue.

Stopping Means Feeling Good
Instead Of Feeling Full

It is good to be full of pleasure instead of full of ice cream. It really helps to think of the food in the past even when it is still in the present and to say out loud, or even to yourself, as you pause for a moment, "This has been great. I have really enjoyed it."

Worrying About Waste

Something gets in the way of learning to stop when we first try it. It's the idea that something terrible will happen if you don't eat everything on your plate!

What's so terrible? The food will be wasted! This belief has been drummed into us from childhood. Many of us eat what other people leave, just because it will be wasted if we don't.

Example:

Jonathan's wife, a natural eater, would quietly transfer what she didn't want over to his plate and he would eat it. One night, as she did this, he said, "No thanks, I don't want it." She was surprised, and said, "But you mustn't waste it. I cooked it." He said, "Well, will you eat it?" She said, "No, I can't. I don't have room." He said, "Well, neither do I."

She was annoyed that some of the food she had cooked would be wasted, even though it was not helping Jonathan to act as the garbage can. Once Jonathan ate it, the food was gone anyway, so it made no difference into which garbage can it went. Nothing terrible would happen if he left it. He resolved the problem by saying, "Put it away in the fridge and I'll have it for lunch tomorrow." He ended up with a couple of tasty lunches and lots of leftovers, and once the latter had grown moss, he threw them out.

When are we wasting food? Unnatural eaters give themselves the "don't waste food" instruction for two reasons: to conserve food, and to continue to have the taste a while longer. You can have the taste by savoring it when you stop, and by enjoying every mouthful. Now we need a way to work on what to do about the waste.

A New Way To Think About Waste

It is logical to believe that we should waste nothing. For some, this belief probably stems from the eras of the Great Depression and wartime, when resources were scarce and we were taught to treasure every morsel. These days, most of us have the opposite problem: too much available food. Yet we fear that something bad will happen if food is not consumed. Food is an organic product. Science tells us that it is impossible to make matter disappear altogether. It just changes in form.

Think about what *really* happens to food. When we eat it, some of it is consumed by the body, but the remainder becomes a waste product that takes a lot of expensive treatment before it can be turned into fertilizer. Some communities send it out to sea. We hear horrendous stories of diseases caused by sewage contaminating the water supply. Food that is not eaten is much easier to recycle into something useful. If you hate to see it go into the garbage, consider composting. There are containers sold today that allow smell-free composting, even in an apartment kitchen. Give the finished product to gardener friends for a present, and see them smile! Or use it for repotting your indoor plants.

Farmers and country people know how useful scraps can be in feeding chickens and pigs. Dog and cat owners can put leftovers to use just by scraping them into a pet's food dish. You can probably come up with even more creative ways. Remember that a healthy supper's leftovers can make a delightful treat for next day's lunch, especially if it's a favorite. Why take a frozen dinner to the company microwave, when you can zap homemade lasagna?

The other option for recycling is to send the extra food through your digestive system—mouth, esophagus, stomach, large and small intestines—with unnecessary strain on the liver, gall bladder, and pancreas as well. Why wear out your body's machinery with this time-consuming process when your brain can come up with so many useful alternatives? You are simply feeding your town's septic or sewer system. Though you might not have thought about it this way, it's probably *more* wasteful to use up extra body energy, water, and pollution-control devices by overeating and digesting than to recycle food any other way.

More About How To Stop

It is OK to leave something on the plate if you don't need it. Children often do this, but we train them out of it (and into unnatural eating) as fast as we can, more to satisfy our own needs than theirs. We want to know that they have eaten enough to be healthy and strong, whether

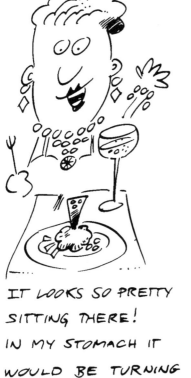

IT LOOKS SO PRETTY
SITTING THERE!
IN MY STOMACH IT
WOULD BE TURNING
INTO BIO DEGRADABLE
MATTER!

they are hungry or not! They are considering the state of their stomachs and what they like to eat; we want them to eat because it is important to us. In the process, we are setting up unnatural behaviors towards food. It is time to stop the cycle!

Go Slow, Stop Halfway

Feel good about leaving something on the plate. Most of us have a hard time with this. Usually you sit down to eat something delicious. The first bites taste superb. You eat quickly, enjoying what you eat. As you see the last bites coming up, you regret that this experience is coming to an end. You clean up the last morsels, somehow getting more pleasure out of those last tastes than from the middle part of the experience, when perhaps you hurried things a bit. You know that it would have been possible to get more pleasure out of the dish if you had taken more time eating it, and then regret that it's all gone. No way could you have left any—it would have been too painful!

This is a fairly typical picture of a person who uses unnatural eating behaviors. A different approach can help you to enjoy what you eat more, and yet feel happy about leaving some on the plate if your stomach is satisfied.

Start

Get in touch with how your stomach feels, and make sure that it has room for what you plan to eat. Your stomach barometer may not be on "hungry," but it should at least be on "empty." At the very least, it needs to have some room left.

Select

Choose the foods that jump your stomach's hurdles best.

Taste

Taste and savor the first few bites. They satisfy not only your hunger but also your taste buds.

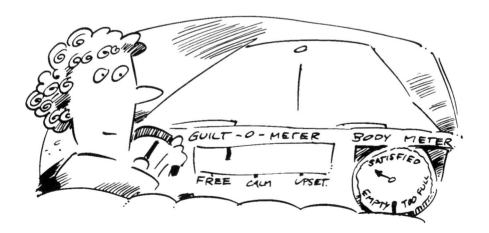

Stop halfway. As you see that you have eaten about half of the dish, *pause.*

Test out your stomach for satisfaction.

How many more bites does it need? Is it satisfied already? Which are the tastiest morsels left?

Decide what of the rest you will eat.

Eat just what you need of the rest, as though each bite were the last one on the plate. You'll find these last bites much more interesting and satisfying than what you used to scrape from the plate at the end.

Keep thinking about how many more bites you really need to fill your stomach, and how many you can happily leave. If you know your stomach doesn't need any more, but you want a bite for your mouth, go ahead and have it and then leave the rest.

Using this behavior, you will find that you get maximum enjoyment from all of your experiences with food, while learning to take note of your body signals and stop when you need to without feeling deprived. Your stomach will feel comfortable rather than bloated, you will feel satisfied with your behavior. Your stomach will be looking after your weight while you enjoy yourself to the fullest!

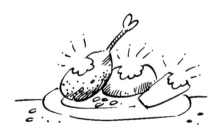

The Balloon Test

Buy a balloon—an ordinary round one, uninflated. Blow the balloon up until it is about as big as your fist. Your stomach is about this size. Hold the balloon in front of your abdomen. Can you imagine something that large inside you? It looks as though it will fit OK. Press your hand on it. Feel the softness of the balloon, and imagine the pressure inside it.

Now blow it up to what you think the volume of food is after you had eaten a large dinner, say at Christmas or Thanksgiving. Hold it against you. How does that look? Comfortable? Can you feel the pressure inside it? How is your "stomach" feeling?

Think of the balloon full of different foods. How would a balloon full of lettuce feel? What about a balloon full of chocolate? Or fries? Or ice cream? Or cheese? Or apple? They feel quite different, don't they?

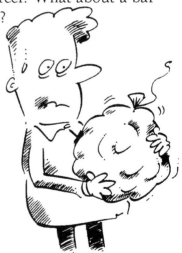

Start practicing now. For the next 24 hours, every time you look at food, try these exercises:

Compare the volume of the food on your plate, in a serving bowl, in a grocery store or restaurant display, with your fist. If you removed some of the liquid, how much would fit comfortably in that volume? That's all your stomach really needs to be satisfied.

WELL, IT WAS LOVELY WHILE I WAS EATING IT !!

Look more closely at the composition of the food. Which parts of it would you really want in your stomach, and which parts would also satisfy your mouth? Which parts could you leave without too much angst? How much of this dish could you eat and leave room for something else that you might enjoy later? Keep remembering your fist-size balloon.

Estimate the number of bites in a food item. This works especially for things like candy bars, croissants, hamburgers, ice cream cones. If the item could be divided into, say, eight bites, how many would your stomach be satisfied with? Can you live with the idea that you are free to eat the item, as long as you accept the responsibility for deciding how many bites you need to satisfy your mouth? (Your fun/enjoyment need.)

How It Works

The first day that I started natural eating, it went well until I remembered that I was giving an after-dinner talk to a group of educators at a club renowned for its huge meals. I began to panic! Then I thought, "Nobody can make me eat that whole dinner. If I want to stick to natural eating, I will eat just enough of each course so that I feel good." The dinner started with a seafood cocktail, so I ate about half of it. Then came the main course, a huge turkey dinner loaded with all the trimmings. I thought about the state of my stomach. At that point it was feeling quite good. I stopped and looked at the plate. I compared the food there to the space I thought was left in my stomach. I said (out loud) "I think my stomach needs about a sixth of this," and ate just that much.

I had to cope with looking at the remaining food for what felt like a long time, then with the waiter asking "Have you finished, madam?" That was not terribly difficult. He would be paid whether I ate it or not. Dessert was Black Forest cake, and I ate about three mouthfuls.

The lady sitting next to me, who was perhaps even a little larger than I was at that time, ate all the seafood, plowed through the whole of the main course, then virtuously gave away her dessert. She looked and spoke longingly about wanting to eat it but was "being good." I gave my talk, and went home satisfied that I had enjoyed the meal. I'm sure that she went home and wolfed down something extra because she was feeling deprived about not allowing herself to eat what "normal" people were able to eat, and what she really wanted all along. That is what I would have done once. I knew exactly how she was feeling.

Try these skills at every meal or snack. Start living your life now not in the future. Work out how your body feels *now*. Enjoy what you are eating *now*. If your stomach feels satisfied, and is likely to be OK for the next hour, don't put anything more in your mouth. Just tell yourself that something else will turn up.

Tip:

While you are learning the stopping process and the thoughts associated with it, serve yourself or order the same size amounts of food you normally would eat. Some people think that they can learn to limit their eating by using a smaller plate or cutting their serving size in half. This method does not allow you to get used to the idea that your stomach, rather than your brain, needs to limit how much you eat rather than your brain. Sooner or later you will be faced with a situation where there is more on your plate (or in an ice cream cone or a candy bar) than your stomach needs. Your brain must learn to:

- Assess the size and appeal of a meal or an item of food
- Consult your stomach for information on how much of the meal you will want

If you always limit the amount of the serving *before* you sit down to eat it, you won't be training your brain! Your brain needs to get used to seeing something left on the plate or thrown away as a normal event, not as something to be concerned about. This will not happen if you continue to eat everything in front of you because the amount is already reduced. That will only reinforce the idea that you must clean your plate—an idea that cramps your sense of freedom.

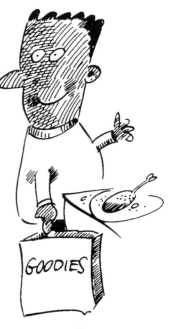

Tip:

Put your car, your purse, and your office on your grocery list. Make sure you have something enjoyable available to eat at all times in the car, in your handbag, in the

I CAN STOP NOW BECAUSE EVEN IF I GET HUNGRY, I CAN HAVE SOME GOODIES ANYTIME!

drawer of your desk at work—wherever you are likely to be. That way, when you ask yourself, "Will my stomach feel better if I eat the rest of this food?" You can reassure yourself by thinking, "If I don't eat any more of this, I've got some special cheese at the office, or some really tasty cookies in the car."

It's a lot easier to stop when you are satisfied if you *know* that you are free to have another enjoyable experience as soon as your stomach is ready again. The more you do Nectar eating, the less you find that you need this support food, but knowing that it is there gives you much more freedom to decide about when to stop.

Example:

Karen, who attended a Nectar group, told me how she taught herself to start and stop and, eventually, trust in the future. During her childhood, Karen's family often had only potatoes to eat for dinner. There was no way any of them would leave anything on their plates, and it was not sensible to trust in an unreliable future. She had carried this belief with her for thirty years, even though food was now plentiful. The idea of trusting in the future was, for her, a total revelation. For a year or so, she kept crackers in the car, apples at work, and her refrigerator packed with goodies of all kinds so she could start whenever she was hungry. She used the stopping thoughts she had learned, and over time she gradually came to accept that she would always have enough to eat. She became a natural eater! Her comment to me, when I visited her group, was, "I have a big bone to pick with you. Why didn't you tell me about this thirty years ago—before I spent so much money and agony on diets?"

How Will I Know When I've Made Progress?

You will know you have retrained your brain when you catch yourself doing something that once would have been unthinkable. For me this happened for the first time one morning when I was pouring cereal into a bowl. I was shaking it out, and when there was a small amount in the bottom of the bowl I found myself thinking "That's all I'll need." I did a double take, and looked again. The amount was about the same as the diets used to tell me to have—a bit less than half a cup.

The change was in what I had *thought*. The thought "That's all I'll need," left me feeling satisfied. Compare it to the old thought, "That's all I am allowed to have," which left me feeling deprived. Outwardly, the behavior was exactly the same. The change was inside me! My thinking and feeling were operating!

You can make little changes, every day, without giving up anything except uncomfortable feelings, by stopping just short of eating it all. Small numbers of calories, over time, add up. That's how people get fat, by eating just a few too many every day. So it will operate the same way in the opposite direction. It won't be fast, but gradually, over time, your body will adjust itself to your natural eating pattern and return to its natural weight—and it will stay there. The behaviors you develop will keep your body healthy and nourished according to its needs.

Some Stopping Thoughts:

- What level is my hunger now, on a scale of 1 to 10?
- If I eat more of this, will my stomach feel better?
- Which are the tastiest bits left? I'll eat those next and review what is left after that.
- Do I feel happy to leave the rest?
- Do I want the wasted bits to go through me first?
- If I leave this, I can always eat the rest any time I like and enjoy it then—in five minutes, ten minutes, or tomorrow.
- How long do I want this meal to last? When do I want to be hungry again?
- Have I eaten a fistful? How full is my balloon?
- Do I need to leave some of this and keep room for something else?
- If I eat the rest and feel overfull, will my stomach feel good?
- I've got some treats in the car for later!

Chapter 12

COPING
WITH THE EXPECTATIONS
OF OTHERS

Once you open the door and pass through into Nectar territory, you will also need to be able to deal with the people who are still out there in Unnatural-Eaters Land. The ideas and beliefs that have caused you and me so many problems are the result of society's best thinking to date. The fact that there is a better way to think is something that will take a while to sink in and become widespread.

It isn't easy to explain Nectar concepts quickly to others because the changes you are experiencing amount to a whole new way of life, based on a whole complex of new ideas. When the family sees you pigging out on something that used to be forbidden, they will probably, out of the goodness of their hearts and because they love you, suggest that maybe you shouldn't be eating it. When you leave food, they are likely to worry that you didn't like it or that it is being wasted. These are old ideas that you've left behind. One of the best ways to help your loved ones to understand is to have them read this book!

But I Love You The Way You Are

In some cases, you may even find that a relationship depends on your being fat. A number of books go into the reasons why it is more comfortable for one person in a relationship to remain overweight; it means that others will not have to change their behavior.

On the other hand, being fat could be used as an explanation or excuse for difficulties in a relationship. For example, a couple may blame a man's inability to have sex with a woman on her appearance, whereas the reason may be much more complex. Appearance is just an easy, uncomplicated thing to blame. If you believe that this is a problem in one or more of your relationships, you might consider seeking counseling assistance (for books on relationships, refer to the reading list in the back of this book).

Here are strategies to help you cope with the common behaviors you are sure to encounter in the people around you as they observe your new way of living.

Situation:

A waiter or waitress in the restaurant looks askance at what you order. Maybe you've decided to have dessert first, and not order anything more until you decide whether you are satisfied! Or, he or she may act surprised at the amount of food you leave on your plate. "Have you finished, madam?"

Solution:

Say to yourself, "Who is paying?" Instead of interpreting what they do as a reflection on you, see it as misguided thought and poor-quality service. Or, try to see the humor in the situation: expect a waiter to be surprised at your requests and try to guess at what will surprise him most. Then smile at your inside joke when he fulfills your expectation. You have befuddled a pro! Now that you have his attention, make sure he understands your order, so you get what you want.

Practice asking for exactly what you want on the menu, rather than what you think the waiter or waitress wants you to have. And make sure that you are clear about when the food should be delivered, if you decide you want to mix up the courses to please yourself. If you want dessert when the others are having soup, make enough noise to ensure that you get it. You don't have to be nasty, just firm and certain that you know you have a right to service. Give a sweet smile and say, "Thank you, yes. That's exactly what I want. I'm sure a good waiter like you can supply it."

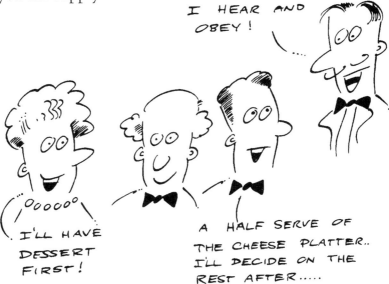

Some other things natural eaters say in restaurants:

· I've already eaten, but I would really enjoy keeping you company while you eat. I'll have more
  time to talk!
· I think I'll just order an appetizer. The main
  courses here are too large for me. I want some
  room for sweets.
· All I really want is the dessert. I'm going to order
  just that, and have it while you have your main
  course.
· I'm going to ask them to pack the rest in a doggie
  bag for me so that I can enjoy it when I'm
  hungry.

Situation:

Someone close to you has made
you a special treat. How can
you refuse it? The person is really trying to please you.

As one man asked me:
"How can I say no to my
mother's chocolate fudge layer
cake? She makes it specially
for me when I go to visit because she knows I like it so
much! My doctor has told me
not to eat it, but it's really hard
to resist her. And then she kind
of forces another piece on me—
she twists my arm."

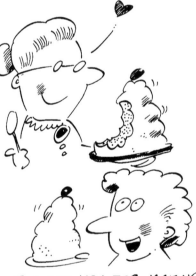

I LOVE YOU FOR MAKING
THIS FOR ME MOM!
COULD I POSSIBLY
TAKE IT HOME?

Solutions:

Appeal to Mom for help. Say, "Mom, I know you made the cake specially for me because you care about pleasing me. And I love you for it. I would like to have just as much of it as my stomach needs right now, and then can I take some home for when I become hungry again? That way I can enjoy it twice!" Then make a big fuss over just how great the two or three bites that you take taste, and how kind she is for pleasing you.

Be a "noisy eater!" Make the noise with your voice instead of your teeth. Make a big noise about how great the food tastes, how much trouble the person has taken, how good you feel about what you have eaten, how "full" you feel, how little room you have left to fit in another morsel. Ask for the recipe, ask for some to take home (you may or may not want it later, it's up to you). What you really are is an *expressive eater*, fulfilling all your needs at once (love, power, fun and especially freedom and survival).

Some of the things you hear natural eaters say in this situation are:

- It sounds/smells delicious, but I'm not hungry right now. Could I eat a little later?
- I couldn't eat another bite.
- You always make wonderful _____. What is your secret?
- What a shame! It looks superb, but I just don't have room. Could I have some to take home?
- I could only fit in a couple of bites. If you don't want to waste it, give me a very small portion.

· That looks and smells wonderful. I wish I had room for it. Could you let me have the recipe?

This is Nectar talk—the language of someone whose body is giving signals about what and how much food to eat, and who is listening to those signals and choosing effective eating behavior.

Exercise:

Think of a situation, perhaps at a party, work or upcoming holiday, where you are likely to encounter food prepared by a friend or relative. Work out something to say that will help you to stick to eating by your own body signals and still keep things comfortable for everyone. Look at the Nectar-talk examples above, and work out where each one could be of use. A good format for a Nectar-talk remark would be:

· A compliment to the cook
· A statement beginning with "but" that describes your physical feeling
· A suggestion about how you could enjoy the food later when you are hungry

Situation:

Someone really disapproves of what you are eating and tells you so.

This person sees you as having a weight problem, and is genuinely trying to help you lose weight by suggesting that what you are eating is bad for you. This person may have no idea of your previous eating habits, especially if you were a "closet eater," eating when there is no one to see you. What you are doing now is "coming out of the cupboard" and eating what you want in public. It's difficult for the people close to you to accept this. What you need is an explanation of what you are doing.

Solution:

Try this: "I am working on a whole new approach to eating, because dieting has always meant putting the weight back on. I am training myself to make all foods equal in my mind, so that eventually I can trust my body to tell me what it needs."

Another solution:

Avoid eating *with* or *in front of* such a person until you've had a chance to focus on your own natural eating process. Then try it out. When they do comment (and they will), let them know that you appreciate their care and concern for you, and ask for their help. Tell them the best way they can help is by not commenting on what you are eating or even whether you have lost weight, because the weight loss will be slow, and you are trying to feel as good as possible about yourself right now. The payoff for them will be that you will be easier to live with—calmer, happier and more satisfied. If this is difficult to do, I am providing you here with a short letter which you could ask them to read.

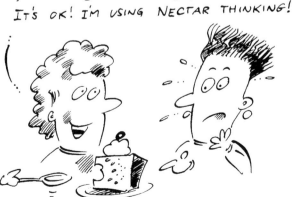

A Letter To My Loved Ones

As you probably know, I have tried many times before to lose weight by dieting. From another person's viewpoint, the problem may appear to be a lack of willpower or motivation. If this were all it is, I would still not be having problems. Although you may not have realized it, I have spent a lot of time criticizing myself because of my eating habits, and feeling bad about them.

This time, I am attempting something totally different. It's called Nectar, and it's a program that I believe offers me more hope than anything else I have attempted in my battle with weight.

Nectar is based on changing my *thinking* about eating. Instead of dieting or overeating, I am learning to use food for its true and primary purpose to satisfy hunger. I will be eating when I am hungry and stopping when I am satisfied. This probably sounds simple, but actually, it means thinking hard and focusing on my thought process when I eat.

I will not be dieting. I will not lose weight quickly (look for changes in six months!) I am aiming at lifelong freedom from weight and eating problems.

What you will see me doing is this:

- Making sure I have an inexhaustible supply of foods that formerly were "forbidden." This helps me think of them as less important so that I can stop focusing on them.
- Eating whatever I want whenever I feel physically hungry, and eating just enough to feel satisfied, and leaving the rest.

- Acting on the urge to eat when not hungry by nurturing myself (with food if necessary) until I learn other ways to think.
- Eating at unusual times or in unusual patterns. I might eat a dessert for breakfast or at the beginning of a meal. I will be unconventional.

I don't expect this to be easy, but if I can relearn my approach to food, my body will eventually reach its proper weight without my dieting. I know your concern stems from the fact that you care about me, and I appreciate that. However, I will receive most help from positive rather than negative comments on what I am doing, and I won't be looking for comments about losing weight.

Rather, it would help if you don't worry about what or when I am eating or when, and allow me to keep you company at mealtimes so that I only eat when I am hungry. I am attempting to learn to think differently so that I can be free from concentrating on food and become a happier person.

Eventually I will be able to arrange to get hungry at mealtimes, but for now I would like to eat only when I need to. For many people like me, Nectar will provide a way of breaking the eating patterns that have caused my weight problems.

Thanks for being open-minded. Your support will help me a lot.

Love,

Thinking Lifelong

One of the Nectar principles is "Think lifelong." The strategies I have mentioned so far are designed to help you to begin to practice and develop natural eating habits.

For a behavior to become a habit that lasts a lifetime, it has to be more need-satisfying than the habits you used to have. All of the skills you will learn will give you freedom and fun. When you were dieting, you used to satisfy your power need by telling yourself that you were good, watching your weight go down, and taking pride in a thinner body. When you are practicing Nectar skills, your power comes from knowing that you are really doing right by your body and living in the pleasant present. Soon the behaviors you learn will feel so natural that you won't think you are doing anything all that different from what you did before. As your beliefs change, your new behaviors begin to feel ordinary—which they are to natural eaters!

I have given you a number of strategies that will help you fill your need for love and belonging in ways other than eating with the family at their mealtimes. You will be feeling so much better, and you should be easier to live with. And, when you understand that people choose their behavior, it gives you a new, positive outlook on life.

Customizing Nectar

These new habits can become lifelong only if they fit in with your lifestyle. Nectar needs to be "made to measure" just right for each person. Here's how some Nectar graduates did it.

Example:

Sarah told me that the most satisfying time of her day was the time after she got the children off to school, when she could sit quietly and have a cup of tea and toast and read the paper—it was her most precious experience. But she wanted the tea and toast even when she wasn't hungry!

Solution:

I told her that under no circumstances should she give that up! If I asked her to do something else less need-satisfying, Sarah would feel that her freedom and fun needs were being abused. So, even if she didn't have a hunger signal at that time, it was important that she have her tea and toast. I suggested, however, that she might start observing her "stopping" signal to decide just how much toast she needed, or take note of how long the tea and toast lasted before she needed to eat again.

Example:

Elizabeth believed that she needed to eat at six o'clock every evening. Even when she was full, it was a routine, and she enjoyed it.

Solution:

Do what you enjoy! It makes sense to plan ahead for a fixed eating time. Giving your body food at intervals so that it gets hungry at the time you plan to eat dinner. If dinner at six or toast at ten is important to you, then keep doing it even if you are not hungry. All you need to do is to work out when your body wants to stop eating.

What helped Elizabeth was thinking about her stomach. She thought about what greasy foods would do in there. She imagined little people pushing trolleys full of raw materials round her stomach factory, slipping over in the grease, cursing the supplier for giving them too much. So she still ate at six o'clock, but she used her new Nectar skills to *select* what she ate and to stop before she was stuffed. As she went on, she noticed her clothing getting looser. Just as we got to the end of the group, she went to the doctor and he weighed her—so she really did still exist, and there was less of her!

Questions And Answers About Nectar

Question:

Do I have to exercise as part of Nectar?

Answer:

Nectar is all about freedom of choice, so it does not prescribe anything! There is no doubt that moderate, aerobic exercise promotes good health and longer life. I won't go into all the reasons, but tons of research supports this. In Nectar, beliefs and thoughts that you have about why you exercise are what matters. Like eating, exercise should be something you do because it helps you to feel good, rather than to lose weight. If losing weight is the only reason why you exercise, then when you have taken off the weight you will stop. If you are aiming for a permanent lifestyle, do it to feel good.

You can become positively addicted to physical activities that you do for about half an hour every day. These exercises get your circulation going and let your mind relax at the same time. Your brain actually releases pleasure chemicals that give you a natural "high." I get one when I leave the swimming pool. I swim as often as I possibly can, for half an hour nonstop. Not fast, just continuously. It's not always easy to convince myself that I should start, but then when I think of how I will feel when I finish, I know that it will be worth it. And if I choose not to go, I definitely feel "down" because I have missed out.

Exercise is need-satisfying for me. When I do it, I feel good. I am not thinking about the mythical future when I might be thinner, I am enjoying the feeling of

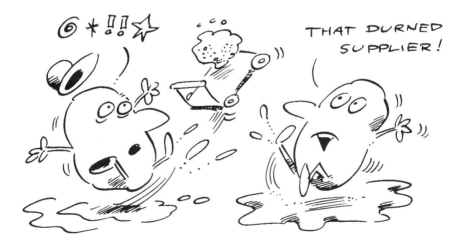

pleasure right now. So, exercise will be a lifelong commitment. I might change the form of exercise depending on my circumstances. For example, if there is no place available to swim, I might walk instead. Or sometimes it might be more need-satisfying to keep someone company in some other form of exercise, such as golf or tennis, so that I am meeting my belonging need as well as my fun and survival needs (mind you, my power need might suffer in golf!).

Question:

Am I doing Nectar right?

Answer:

Most people feel more accomplished and meet their power needs if they can be sure they are doing Nectar "right." You won't have any simple yardstick such as scales. So, how will you know if it's working? Nectar's aim is for your new behaviors to feel so natural that you *feel* as though you are eating as much as you ever did.

When Nectar is working, you are enjoying yourself more, but somehow the weight has decided to fall away. This is what happened for me. It seemed almost criminal to be able to have such a good time around food and find that my clothing was getting looser!

Question:

When can I expect results?

Answer:

It takes time—more for some, less for others. I started to notice changes in my body at around the eight-week mark, and I was the first of our group to see things actually happening. For Jenny, they started to happen almost six months after she started this method of being around food. Twelve months later, she looks and feels very different. It happened that way for most of the other people in this experimental group. We started in May, 1992. Fifteen months later, we were all thinner and eating more naturally.

Tip:

One way to recognize how much your beliefs have changed is to find someone who is still in diet mode, and listen to what she says. Remember when you used to think that way? How painful it was!

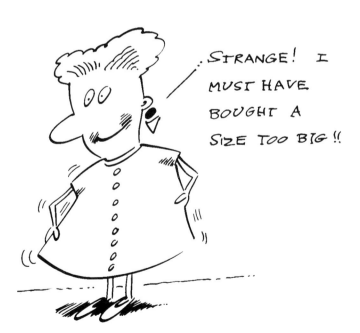

STRANGE! I MUST HAVE BOUGHT A SIZE TOO BIG!!

Check-In Questions

- When you need a treat, can you give yourself permission, and find something that you really enjoy?
- If you have a binge now and then, does it last as long as it used to?
- Can you remember the "stuffed" feeling you used to have when you overate? How long has it been since that happened?
- Have you come across former binge foods that you had forgotten about?
- Have you caught yourself doing something that would have been unthinkable before you learned these new ideas?

If you can answer yes to any of these questions, you are on the right track. You will probably be able to say yes to more than one!

Example:

Lorelei tells the story of some lamb chops. She was in the supermarket. The lamb chops are packaged in threes. Usually she buys two packets so she and her husband can each have two, and she puts the others away in the freezer. This day, she stopped at the meat display and was moving on when she looked down and saw that she had put only *one* packet of lamb chops in her cart. Automatically, she had thought, "That'll be enough—two for him and one for me!" Her brain had readjusted to her new Nectar eating patterns so that she was naturally limiting what she bought, with no feelings of deprivation or guilt, no "shoulds" or "shouldn'ts," just an acceptance of a normal state of affairs.

Question:

At one time or another, as you are learning Nectar or thinking long term, you're bound to say to yourself, "It's not fair! Why should I have to make my body limit my eating when other people don't? If I only eat what my body wants, I'll still have to give up eating lots of desirable foods because I'm not hungry!" That's how I would be thinking (and feeling deprived) at this point in the process. It doesn't feel fair!

Answer:

Show me the decree that says life has to be fair! People can act fair or not fair, but life has a way of doing whatever it wants. If the body you have inherited and developed needs less food than someone else's body, then that's the way life is. Maybe life is fair to you in other ways.

You don't have to give up eating lots of delectable things! You *can* have lots and lots of wonderful, pleasurable experiences with food, with no guilt and no weight gain, once you learn to feel satisfied with less—once you learn *stopping*. No food is off limits to you if you stop as soon as you've had enough. Think to yourself, "Everything that passes my lips should be a pleasurable experience." Don't fill up your stomach with food that you don't like or don't want.

Example:

Laurie reported that once she stopped watching what others ate and took her focus off food, she began really enjoying the company of her friends and family far more. Somehow, by thinking about them instead of food, she

satisfied her belonging and fun needs far more than she
had with eating.

Question:

This is so hard! Why is it taking so long?

Answer:

It will get easier. If your body has gone into "famine"
mode because of the way you have been dieting (alter-
nately denying it for a period and then overfeeding it), it
probably will need only small amounts of food at first,
because it has learned to conserve everything you put
into it. But once it gets used to being fed whenever it
sends a signal, it will gradually start to act naturally and
ask for more. For instance, you may find that the first
time you wait for a hunger signal, it takes forever! But as
your body becomes accustomed to this method of eating,
it is quite likely to become hungry around mealtimes
(surprise!). You will eventually know how your body will
react to certain types and amounts of food. You will be
able to plan getting hungry just when you want to.

Question:

How much weight will I lose?

Answer:

Your body will take itself back to whatever is the weight
at which it feels best. Be aware that this may or may not
agree with the picture in your head of how you should
look. Remember that models these days are very under-
weight, which is no more healthy than being overweight.
You don't know what they might be doing to their bodies

to keep them that way; there could be a lot of agony under that beautiful outside. Trust your body to know what it wants and you will start to look and feel happier!

Question:

I'm feeling impatient. When will I see results?

Answer:

Start living your life in the pleasant present, not in the future perfect. Settle for enjoying what you are eating *now*. Check in with your body and see how it feels *now*. If it feels satisfied, and likely to be OK for the next hour, don't put anything more in your mouth. Just tell yourself that something else will turn up.

Tip:

Again, my way of feeling comfortable about not eating all of whatever I select is to make sure that I have something enjoyable to eat available at all times (in the car, in my handbag, in the drawer of my desk) wherever I am likely to be. That way, when I ask myself, "Will my stomach feel better if I eat the remainder of this?", I feel much more freedom when I answer no. The more you do Nectar, the less you'll need this support food, but knowing that it is there gives you much more freedom to decide when to stop eating.

Tip:

Many foods actually look better than they taste. Having pleasurable experiences with food doesn't necessarily mean eating. Sometimes all you need to do is to visit a bakery, enjoy the lovely displays and smells, ooh and aah, pick out something that appeals to you, and buy it. Later, when you examine what you really want, it might not be what you wanted after all. But you satisfied your fun and freedom needs.

Example:

Wendy reported that when she started the program and wanted to make friends with enemy foods, she went out and bought a box of chocolates. This seemed to be what everybody else was talking about, so they must be what she should get. When she got them home, ate one, and really focused on its taste, she found that she didn't even really like them! All she liked was the idea of chocolates.

Sue, on the other hand, was a chocolate-cookie freak. The richer, the better. Sue loved them. But after about four weeks of having them available all the time, she reported that the open packet had remained in the cupboard all week. She still enjoyed them but didn't need them all, or all the time. She found herself choosing boring foods like boiled eggs because that was what her body started telling her it wanted.

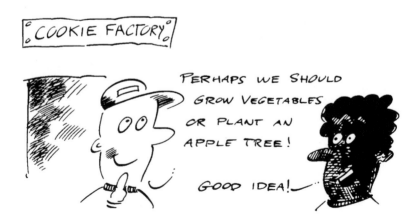

Question:

What will people think if I eat at odd times?

Answer:

Worrying about what people think can be a terrible distraction from focusing on what *you* think. It restricts you in all sorts of ways, not only in relation to eating. We all have pictures in our heads of how we want other people to view us. But if you stop worrying so much about what *others* think, you will reduce the power they have in controlling your life and experience enormous freedom!

The Myth Of Three Square Meals

We live in a society in which *when* you eat, *where* you eat, and *what* you eat are thoroughly and subtly cued by customs. You will be bucking the trend of what, where, and when as you adopt Nectar training. You will be developing your own customs. But be prepared if the rest of the world balks! For example, we are conditioned to think of three meals a day as being the routine we should follow, whether we are hungry or not. Probably the three meals idea grew up because it boosts the energy levels to put something in our stomachs when they are empty. Quite sensible.

But when you start thinking of what we have done to this custom, it boggles the mind. For a real dinner, we may have soup, appetizer, entree, main course, dessert, after-dinner items, wines appropriate for each type of food, and sorbets to clear the palate. What an appetizer does other than *take away* the appetite I am really not sure! I know it is supposed to prepare you to eat more. (Increase your appetite? Give you more psychological signals to eat more? What a useful idea!)

Example:

A young woman who is a natural eater was discussing this with me a couple of days ago. She told of her early experience in her family, where her mother brought her up as a natural eater. The food was placed in the center of the table, and she was encouraged to eat the amount she needed. She never heard about the starving children and was never told to clean her plate. Food and eating were never a big deal.

She told me a terrific story about her mother who is also a natural eater, slim and elegant. One evening her mother went to a banquet where there were many courses. She has a sweet tooth, so she had dessert for every course—six desserts! She said that they looked so good that she wanted to sample them all. And sample them is what she did. She ate only a little of each and had a wonderful time!

Maximum enjoyment, no thoughts about weight or what people will think—this is natural eating at its purest! Of course, a meal like this does leave things like vitamins and health a little out of consideration. But the secret is that it's not difficult to maintain a healthful balance overall. With freedom to choose whatever you want, it often turns out that what you want is something that helps your body feel healthy. It is more healthy to eat just enough of what you really want instead of plowing through all the courses.

Situation:

What will people think if I eat when I am hungry at work instead of at my conventional lunch time? I hate the idea that people who see me eating at my desk will think I am a terrible pig. They'll think, "She eats *all the time!*"

Solution:

People who smoke think nothing of having a break for a cigarette. Why should having a break for a short meal be any different? This brings up the question of breaks at work. Many people feel uncomfortable about having a break without eating or drinking or smoking, as though it is not right to have a break just because you need some time away from the work. We are conditioned to feeling somehow that we are unusual if we choose to just sit and talk, read a book or the newspaper, or go for a walk. Obeying the unwritten rule, or even making up the rule, can be a way for people to establish some power for

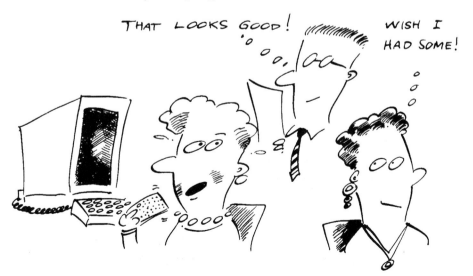

themselves if they are working in a crummy job that gives them little satisfaction. Allow your body to have more say in what you do rather than relying on what people might think.

Situation:

You may have to cope with that little voice inside that says, "I can't do that. I'm too fat." Many overweight people will not go swimming or appear on the beach unless they are covered from head to foot. "I can't let people see me like this," they think. Or they might refrain from playing volleyball or other fun games with friends. They might even reject the idea of going to a private gym.

Solution:

Just think about your own thought patterns when you see a very overweight person with the courage to turn out in a swimsuit or go in for some sport. You might think, "Boy, that person is fat!" If you don't have a weight problem you stop there. The next thought might be, "I'm glad I'm not that big!"

What damage does this do to the person in the swimsuit? Absolutely none! In fact, he or she has helped a couple of other overweight people to feel better about themselves! Nobody on the beach has ever become sick, desperate, or been hurt in any way, just by looking at someone overweight. Most people are too busy thinking about their own appearance to worry at all about someone who is overweight.

And would any of our friends really like us less if we turned out in a swimsuit? Is our appearance the reason we are friends? If they are real friends, they are with us because we accept each other and enjoy each other's company. You can translate this thinking to many other scenarios, such as wearing particular clothes or bright colors, eating exactly what you want in public, buying what you want.

Situation:

Eating with my family is important, but I'm not hungry at mealtimes.

Solution:

Eventually, you could eat at regular mealtimes with your family. When you are just starting, it is important to get back in touch with the signals your body gives you when it needs to be fed. This will help you move faster along the path to natural eating. Nectar is all about developing a natural eating lifestyle. As you regulate your food consumption to satisfy your hunger, your hunger signals will eventually coincide with mealtimes.

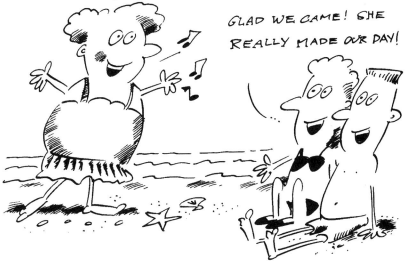

Chapter 13

KID STUFF

How to help your child become a natural eater

When we really examine where we got our beliefs that we shouldn't waste food, that we should always clean our plates, and that a cookie or a candy will make us feel better, we can trace many of them back to our childhood. So will our kids!

If you have been doing your best to be a good parent, chances are that some of the things you have learned in this book are making you squirm. You can now see, as I can, that many of the things we did with our children have trained them out of natural eating behaviors. We probably repeated many of the things our parents did with us. So if you are a parent, and think that these ideas make sense, you may, like me, be feeling guilty about the way you have taught your children to be unnatural eaters. Don't despair! It helps a lot to work out why you did what you did.

How could I have done that to little Susie? There are lots of *good* reasons! First, you wanted your child to be healthy, to eat the foods that you had been told were good for him or her. Second, when you had provided the food, you wanted to know that it had been properly used up— it had not been wasted. There might even have been times when you provided an example by eating what was left yourself. (I call that the old "model garbage disposal" trick.) Third, having put effort into preparing the food, you met your need for achievement when you saw it eaten.

The most critical of these reasons is your child's health. This was the message my mother gave to me, and I passed it on to my family.

By considering their well-being, we were simply doing the best we knew how to be good parents and bring up healthy children. We took notice of doctors' research, nutritionists' advice, the very latest in meal planning for a balanced diet based on four servings of this and six of that from the four basic food groups. We force-fed ourselves and our children quantities of good food. We ignored our stomachs in the process, but the beliefs on which we were acting were the best that society could provide, and they are still prevalent today.

What Can I Do Now?

What you *can* do, if your children are still young, is to help them maintain the connection between hunger and food, so that they grow up to be natural eaters. This means helping them to be aware of what hunger feels like, how much food takes away the hunger, the difference between being hungry in your mouth and being hungry in your tummy, and how different foods feel in your tummy after you have eaten them.

Situation:

Geoffrey comes in about an hour before dinnertime, saying, "Mom, I'm hungry. Can I have a cookie?" Often, Mom's answer is, "No, it will spoil your dinner." What she is thinking is, "If Geoffrey eats a cookie now, he won't eat the vegetables I am cooking for dinner. Vegetables are better for him than cookies, so he shouldn't eat anything right now." If Mom wins, what actually happens is that Geoffrey's brain learns to cope with his hunger signal by forgetting it. He is learning that you eat for reasons other than hunger.

Solution:

A better way to teach Geoffrey about how food affects his body would be to say, "If you are hungry now, and dinner will be ready in an hour, how much food and what kind of food would help you to feel good now and still be hungry at dinner time?" Work out with him what he might try out, and discuss at dinner time whether he made a good choice. Next time the same situation arises, work it out again.

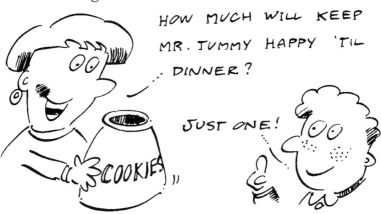

Situation:

I really worry that my four-year-old isn't eating enough! He's never hungry at meal times.

Solution:

Help your child learn what hunger feels like. Some children do not associate the feeling of hunger with the need to eat. These are the ones parents worry about because they just don't eat enough. Help them to identify where the feeling of being hungry comes from in their body, and what kind of food would help. If you are really worried about how your child survives because he or she appears to eat so little, write down everything that the child eats for a couple of days. You will probably find that little Sally or Bobby is grazing rather than eating at mealtimes. Your child may also have an energy-efficient constitution that makes full use of all the food he or she eats.

Tip:

The more relaxed you are about food, the more likely your child will be to select a suitable diet. Monica tried this out. Her friends were horrified when they visited her, finding that she had laid out big bowls of candy, chocolates, chips, and allowed the children to eat whatever they wanted. She said that at first they gorged themselves, but once they found that the treats were always there, they would take just one now and then. It was hard on the visiting children, who might go temporarily haywire, but she did her own children a favor.

I am not recommending that your children live exclusively on ice cream, but it is important to help them equalize food in their minds. Instead of holding up dessert as a reward ("You can't have dessert until you have eaten your vegetables"), work on *hungry* or *not hungry.* What is the feeling in his tummy that says that he doesn't need any more vegetables? If he is not hungry for his vegetables right now, he can put them away for later when he is ready to eat. In these days of microwave ovens, it's not usually a chore to heat things up. If he's not hungry, he's not hungry; dessert shouldn't come into it.

Really, when you think about it, it is a difficult feat to have every person in the family hungry at exactly the same time. Children are behaving quite logically when they say they don't have room for any more, and then get hungry an hour later. The satisfaction signal that they get from their tummy is a really important one, yet we train them to ignore it. It might be better to help them recognize the signal. What does it feel like? How long does it last? What is it telling them? When they say they have room for some ice cream, is that message coming from their mouth or their tummy?

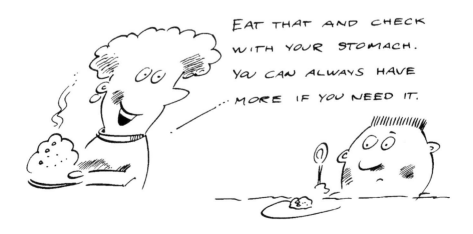

Tip:

Try eating "family style." Instead of putting food on individual plates and expecting everyone to clean them, let the family serve themselves the amount they need. The other option is to make initial portions small and offer seconds, having the occasional discussion of how much more will fill the stomach.

The Overweight Child

No matter how tempting it might be to "help" this way, never put an overweight child on a diet. It will just maintain the problem and teach the child a lot of fat-producing behaviors or even start them on a course towards anorexic or bulimic disorders. A recent study in New South Wales, Australia discovered that children as young as six years of age were beginning to diet! They were setting themselves up for a lifetime of problems with food.

Instead, help overweight children get in touch with their own body signals. Initially, serve them small portions, and train them to think about how much more their stomach needs. Don't restrict them from eating the foods they like, but get them to think about how each food will feel in their stomach and whether it will do a good job of making them feel good. Get them to think of food in terms of bites. Work out how many they need right now, and leave some for later.

Be A Role Model

Let your children know your own healthy attitudes. Food does not solve all problems. Are you always hankering after fast-food ads or chocolate desserts, giving the message that some foods are naughty but nice? Are you giving messages that food is a band-aid? When a child is upset, does he need a cookie or sympathy? Will a cool drink of water do the same job as a cookie? If he is tired, should he eat, or rest? If he is tense, should he eat, or relax? If he is hurting, does he need food, or understanding and time?

Everyone's body is different, and that is OK. You will have to counter the media messages glorifying thin models. One way to introduce this is to stress that many of the people seen on TV and magazine covers are almost unnaturally thin. It's *not* the way everybody looks, and underneath that glamorous appearance there may be someone who stays unhappy and hungry all the time to keep their weight down. For example, it is now becoming more widely known that many models are anorexic or bulimic. Being thin does not automatically lead to happiness. Happiness comes from meeting your needs and balancing your life. You can do that no matter what your appearance is.

Kids Don't Need To Diet

If you start with Nectar principles when your children are young, they should retain the natural eating behaviors they were born with: the sensitivity to body signals, and the ability to choose the foods that suit them. Think about how animals know what foods they need. For example, the koala bear can only eat a certain kind of eucalyptus leaf. Koalas never eat the same foods as dingoes, which are carnivores. They each know what will suit them. So do we! Koalas, I am sure, and hummingbirds too, never think about whether they are too fat or worry about putting on weight. Left to their own devices, they eat what they need and their weight suits them fine. We humans could do ourselves a favor by copying them.

On the other hand, starvation and chronic malnutrition leads to decreased intellectual capacity in children because the body will hoard fat cells and use up protein before it uses all the fat. I know some girls hold a belief that it's not smart to be too smart, but in these feminist days it should be easy enough to counter that argument. If I had a child—especially a teenage daughter—who appeared to be limiting her food intake in an effort to stay thin, I would explain to her that the more she limits her intake of food, the more her body will fight to maintain its weight. Explain that it is not the eating, but the dieting that actually makes us fat in the long run, because we develop so many fat-producing beliefs about food and eating. Teach your children about needs and how to balance them, and give them accurate messages about what, when, and how much to eat. Their appearance will stay at its best if they eat a good, balanced intake of food and exercise regularly.

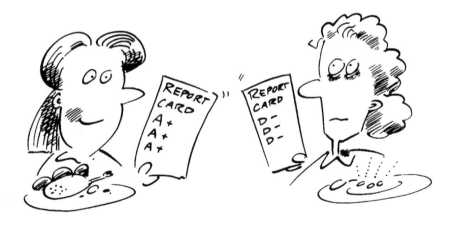

Chapter 14

MORE QUESTIONS AND ANSWERS

Here are some more questions people commonly ask while learning Nectar thinking.

Question:

I still worry when I feel the urge to eat and I know it's my mouth that is hungry, not my stomach. If I do eat then, am I going off Nectar, and wrecking my chances of losing weight? What if I eat when I have a cold, or I am feeling depressed? What should I do when I feel bad?

Answer:

Notice that this question still focuses on weight loss. This is common after dieting for so many years. It just means that your thought processes haven't yet converted completely. Focus instead on giving yourself permission to do what feels right. Tell yourself that if you really need to eat, it's OK. If you have the freedom to eat whatever you want, you will eat less and perhaps next time do something different. The main thing is not to eat blindly. Ask yourself, "What would be the most delicious thing I could eat to really make myself feel good?" Arrange to eat it. You will find that the urge to binge will go away much earlier.

When you feel bad, just give yourself permission to feel bad until you want to feel better. Feeling bad is usually not fatal. Look at your needs: power, freedom, love, and fun. Is there one that you are not meeting? Have a good look at what you really want. Is what you are doing getting you what you want?

No matter what you decide to do or not do, you will do less harm if you relax and have confidence in your body's ability to look after your weight. The more relaxed you are about your need to eat, the less you will need to eat.

Question:

I'm worried about the small amount of food that satisfies my hunger. I don't want to stop eating after so little. Will it be like this forever? Will I ever be able to eat normally?

Answer:

Yes, your body's need for food will change gradually as it reaches its natural weight. While you are overweight, your body needs less food to satisfy it. This is partly because your old dieting behavior may have put it into "famine" mode so that it needs less than normal to survive, or perhaps your body may have a lot of energy stored away in its fat cells. As the reserves deplete, and your body learns that it always gets enough to satisfy it, you will need to eat more food to feel satisfied and you will reach a normal eating pattern. If you ride out your fear, your eating will become normal. Your body will start cooperating with your eating instead of fighting it.

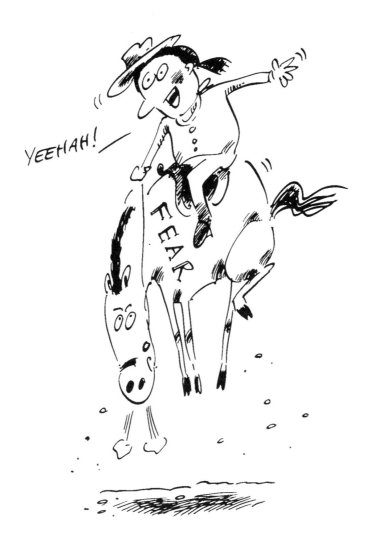

Question:

I am still spending a lot of time thinking about food during this program. Will I ever reach a stage where I don't think about food at all? Isn't this just another "non-diet?" Lots of diets books promise that I won't have to diet. Do you really mean it?

Answer:

In the beginning, you certainly will be paying a lot of attention to food and your beliefs about it. But what you will be thinking about is different. You will be concentrating on answering body signals instead of denying them, feeding your body what it wants instead of feeling constrained by rigid rules about food, believing in yourself as a person instead of feeling controlled by scales. The difference is you will pay attention to your thoughts about food rather than being obsessed by it. The longer you work with these ideas, the more natural your new behavior will feel, and the less you will think about food at all. It will become just a natural part of life, something to enjoy in its place, something you think about when you are hungry.

Question:

If I can eat whatever I want, how will I know that I am eating a balanced diet so that I will be healthy? If my stomach always says "fatty foods," won't I be giving myself other health problems?

Answer:

If you really listen to your stomach and ask it what it wants, you will find that you get answers that are probably not what you expected. Your body will let you know what it needs. When I consult my stomach, oatmeal or tomatoes often feel more appealing than chocolate or fries. Although you may want to binge on one food for some time, over a period you will actually choose a balanced diet. In any case, if you have health reasons for eating in a particular way, you are free to do so, as long as you give yourself as much freedom as possible to enjoy whatever satisfies you. Be as flexible as you can and trust your body to know what it needs. You are in charge! Remember that when people go on a near-starvation diet, they are actually on a diet that is almost exclusively fat— their own fat! How healthy is this?

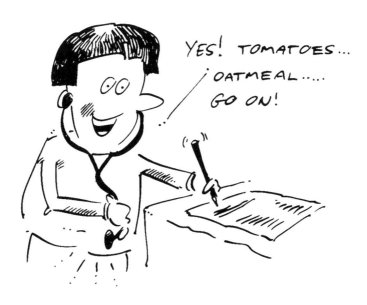

Question:

I am diabetic. How can I be free to eat whatever I want? It's a matter of life and death that I eat certain foods.

Answer:

Clearly, if you have a health problem related to food, you will find it more difficult to feel free to eat whatever you want. I think the only way to get your feeling of freedom while eating what is good for you is to work out what is really going on in your life. Diabetic people often see their condition as a disease that sets them apart from normal eaters. All that has actually happened is that the body, instead of regulating its supply of blood sugar, has passed the job over to the mind, so it has to be done consciously by paying attention to what, when, and how much to eat. This is not easy to accept, and it also is not wise to allow yourself to get really hungry. The more you check in at hurdle number six, and work out what will really feel good in your body, the easier it will be to find that freedom. The one thing you must face is that keeping to a strict diet does not help if you also binge on forbidden foods.

Question:

I really worry that eating whatever I want will lead to an unbalanced diet, even though you tell me my body will work things out.

Answer:

Perhaps you could take a multi-vitamin and mineral supplement as insurance each day. And if you need a lot of fiber, try a large bowl of high-fiber breakfast cereal to keep you regular while you explore what you would really like to eat.

Question:

How am I supposed to feel good about myself if I don't like the way I look?

Answer:

This is certainly a difficult thing to do, but it is the self-criticism about your appearance that creates many of the negative thoughts and feelings which result in overeating for comfort. Whenever you feel a negative thought about yourself coming on, challenge it:

- Is your appearance the *only* thing about you that determines how you feel about yourself?
- Can you start giving yourself credit for the other good things?
- Say to yourself, "I'm not fat because I have more problems than other people. All I have is a set of behaviors which are going to change."
- Say to yourself, "My friends like me because of who I am, not because of how I look."

The more you accept yourself the way you are right now, and live your life in the present, the more likely you are to find that your body becomes healthy and attractive.

Question:

I still want to lose weight. I have been working on my new behaviors for a couple of months and I haven't lost weight. Will it happen?

Answer:

It's difficult to get away from the diet mentality, but if you can relax and allow your body to do its work, the weight will slowly and gradually slip away. You are unlikely to notice big changes quickly. But if you can imagine being free from having to lose weight for the rest of your life, can you give yourself a few months or even a year?

Think of how much more pleasant life is now with Nectar than it was when you were dieting, bingeing, worrying, criticizing yourself. Has your bingeing decreased? Are you eating a bit less than you used to? Get the best out of life in the present as you are, rather than wasting it worrying about the future. If you are using Nectar thinking most of the time, the weight loss *will* happen. If you let go of wanting to be thin, it will just happen naturally. Have confidence in your body—it will return to its natural weight.

Question:

Although I've stopped worrying about losing weight as the main focus in my life, is it OK to still think about it?

Answer:

If you have been thinking these thoughts for a long time, they are firmly embedded in your behavioral system, and naturally they will surface now and then. When they come, just remind yourself of the new Nectar thinking. Habits take time to break.

Question:

How can I tell someone who I think is very overweight about Nectar? What should I say? She is very defensive about diets and about criticism of her size. I am worried about their health and it is difficult to approach her.

Answer:

I think the place to start is to say that you have discovered that being overweight is not the product of problems but of learned behaviors. Maybe you could quote the Minnesota Study. Tell her that Nectar does not aim at weight loss. Its aim is to help you not to gain weight or to worry about your eating, so that you can enjoy food without fear.

Question:

People ask me, "How much have you lost?" I don't know how to answer them.

Answer:

What I say is, "I am not actually trying to lose weight. All I know is that I have lost my weight problem. I plan to weigh myself in June." I'm not saying *which* June.

Question:

I still occasionally weigh myself. I can't seem to throw the scales away. Will this affect my success? I'd like to get rid of my scales, but I can't.

Answer:

It depends a lot on what you *think* when you weigh yourself. If you worry because you have put on a pound or your weight hasn't changed, then you are holding yourself in diet mode. If you are saying to yourself, "I shouldn't be doing this," and feeling a bit furtive about it, then you are probably not doing much harm, as long as you don't let the scales decide what you will do about eating today — and as long as you don't use food to stop the guilt.

Question:

My doctor told me I need to have an operation and that because of my weight, this is dangerous. He told me to lose weight before I have the operation. I'm worried that I won't lose weight in time to have the operation. What should I be doing to solve this problem?

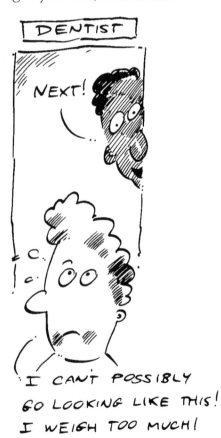

Answer:

This is a special situation. Eat according to your body signals as much as you can, and each time, stop as soon as you are satisfied. You still do not need to weigh yourself. The fat will leave without your knowing how much you weigh. Concentrate on thinking about caring for yourself rather than on losing weight. You might also consider doing some exercise so that you feel good as well. Exercise helps to tone your body.

Question:

Do I really have to leave food, or can I just serve myself less in the first place? Does it really make any difference?

Answer:

Yes, it *does* make a difference! Learning to stop eating when you are satisfied is the behavior that gives you freedom to eat whatever you like. You can't always control how much food is put in front of you, and leaving food is a behavior that we all find really hard to put in place. You will probably find that, at home, your thoughts will automatically limit how much you serve yourself because you will become accustomed to smaller amounts. If you often leave just that last bite or two, you will be much more successful with Nectar.

Question:

My partner is complaining about putting on weight. I can see that the reason for this is because my leftovers and previously forbidden food are being eaten. What should I say?

Answer:

Every person is in charge of his own behavior. You don't actually put the food in your partner's mouth, I presume! You probably need to share your thoughts about stopping and about waste.

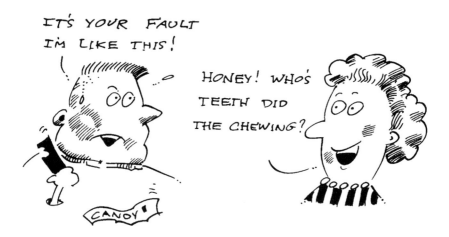

Question:

I still feel the need to eat with my family at dinnertime even when I'm not hungry. I don't want to stay away from them, but when I see them eat I want to eat too! Is this wrong, or how can I deal with it in another way?

Answer:

As you learn to give your body what it needs, you will also be able to get hungry at dinnertime. But even if you are not hungry, and eating with the family is important to you, then go ahead and eat, but work on stopping when you are full. Treat it as an opportunity to learn stopping and leaving some food. If you worry about the example you are setting for the children, I would say that letting them leave some is probably giving them a chance to retain their natural eating behaviors.

Question:

I'm still finding that I binge-eat and, although I realize it isn't happening as often, I was hoping it would disappear altogether. When can I expect this to stop, or am I being unrealistic?

Answer:

This is just the old behaviors resurfacing. The important thing is what you tell yourself when you binge. Treat the urge to binge as a sign that you need to nurture yourself (that's all a binge really is—a way to take care of yourself). Think about what you really need:

- Do you need rest? Then rest!
- Do you need to do something interesting? Find something interesting to do!
- Do you need company? Find a way to talk to someone!

The more you treat the urge to binge as a signal to think and act instead of something you have to fight, the less often it will appear. Give yourself a couple of years before you worry about still feeling that urge to binge.

Question:

Sometimes I can't find a match for my stomach. I feel frustrated because I can't think of anything that will feel good in my stomach. Is this normal? What should I do about it?

Answer:

Yes, that is normal. We have spent so long divorced from the reality of our bodies that it takes time to improve our communication. And your mouth will always remain a big factor in deciding what you want to eat. If your stomach isn't giving you a clear signal, take over the job yourself. Think about what would be good for your body—and eat it!

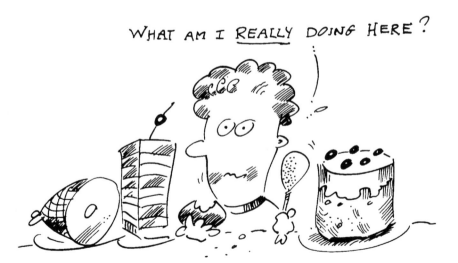

WHAT AM I <u>REALLY</u> DOING HERE?

Chapter 15

PUTTING NECTAR INTO PRACTICE AND GETTING RESULTS

Maybe you've read through this book to the end, liked some of the ideas, tried a few of them, and saw how they worked. But you're not sure whether you really want to jump in with both feet. Or maybe you do but you're not clear how to get started. You love the freedom to choose how to run your life. Here are some options:

You Could Keep On Dieting

One of your options is to put the book away and continue with your dieting. If all you want is to lose a few pounds, and you have never experienced yo-yo weight loss, then go ahead. Just be careful not to allow yourself to become caught up in the dieting thoughts that can cause so much trouble in the future. If you can do this, good luck.

It's going to be a tempting thought to say to yourself, "I'll lose the weight first, then do what she suggests about my thinking." Unfortunately, this thought will lead you right back into the usual dieter's problems. You can take your one chance in twenty that you might make it, if those odds are good enough for you. At the very least, if you fail, you will know that there is nothing to be ashamed of, because you are just one of the majority!

Well, I admit to a little hidden hope that I have spoiled dieting for you, because I know from many years of experience what happens to most of us long term. I wish you all the best!

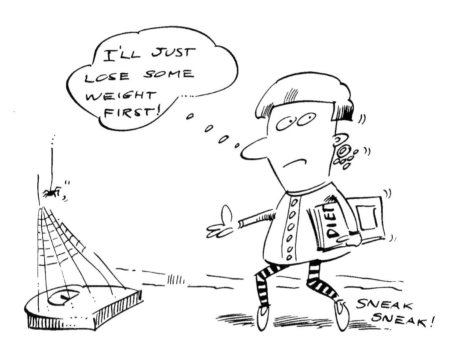

You Could Try Out A Few Nectar Ideas— Have Just A Taste!

Take just a few thoughts that struck you as you read the book, and keep them in mind. Many of the people associated with me in the development of this book have done that, with at least some results. If this is what you choose to do, then without being prescriptive I would like to suggest that you keep in mind the basics:

- You can eat whatever you want as long as it's what you enjoy most.
- Eat what you really want right now.
- All foods should compete for a place in your stomach.
- Stop eating when you feel satisfied rather than when you feel full.

These four key ideas will help you toward the sense of freedom that Nectar can give you. Maybe they will be enough to change your life. If after a while they start feeling really good to you, then you might come back to the book and follow the next suggestion.

Or You Could, As We Aussies Say, Give It A Go!

If you really believe that the thoughts in this book are important enough to take you into a life of real freedom in your eating, and want to use the book to do it, I suggest that you go back and read carefully one chapter a week. Pick out two key thoughts that are important to you personally in that chapter, and learn them. (Write them on a card and carry it with you, or put them where you see them—*not* on the refrigerator!) Practice those thoughts whenever the urge to eat hits you. As those thoughts become more a part of what you think, move on to the next chapter. Emphasize the free nature of this thinking.

If your old dieting thoughts return every now and then, don't panic. That is normal. After all, it took you a long time to learn them, so they will keep coming back from time to time. Just be aware of them and replace them with your new thinking. Perhaps there were some images that particularly made sense to you; bring them back into focus and keep them in the front of your mind.

As you work on Nectar thinking, you will wonder from time to time, "Am I doing it right?" Nectar feels so good that it seems almost wrong to enjoy yourself, and you might start worrying that you will put on weight. Nectar also feels "normal" and "natural" rather than difficult, so you may think you are doing "nothing." Talk to some people who are still dieting, and assess whether your thoughts are different from theirs. Reread the bit in Chapter 5 about the men in Minnesota. Have your ideas changed? Are you bingeing less frequently, or are the binges lasting a shorter time? Are you treating them as opportunities to look after yourself and eat only foods that really feel good?

Sometimes it is difficult to trust your body to look after your weight. Changes will probably be slow, unless you are able to listen really well to your body signals and obey them. In fact, when Jenny did an informal, early follow-up of Nectar graduates in Australia, she found that—guess what—one in twenty of them had lost a lot of weight! You can make a diet out of Nectar if that is what you want. If you are too rigid about body signals, always waiting for hunger signals, always stopping when you are satisfied, continuing to restrict yourself in every way, keeping your focus on food and losing weight, you will loose the essence of the Nectar ideas. But the great majority of the people we contacted had the outcome Nectar aims for: they were feeling free and good about themselves, and food was no longer a worry. Most had lost a little weight three months after they finished the program and their expectation was that it would continue to come off slowly, maybe over the next couple of years. Food, eating, and weight loss were no longer a big deal. I cannot count the number of people I have met who quietly show me a little excess room in the clothes they are wearing and say, "It's coming. It's slow, but it's working, and I feel so great." It is that "great" feeling that lets you know you are doing it right.

Don't worry if at first it is difficult to stop and not have regretful thoughts. We have those thoughts at the end of any pleasurable activity. Regret is much more freeing than "deprived" thoughts. Leaving food is the most difficult part of Nectar, but the positive ideas come with practice.

You Could Read More Of The Literature

Look through the list of suggested readings at the back of the book. These books can give you more understanding of control theory and ways to apply it in your life. Control theory really helps you not to control other people, or even to control yourself, but to *feel* in control of yourself, and to be able to take effective control of your life. You can improve relationships, work through problems, and lead a more fulfilling life.

Nectar Results

You can expect short-term, and long-term results. The short-term results of Nectar thinking are:
- Having fun around food
- Balancing your life
- Feeling assertive and in control
- Enjoying lots of great experiences
- Feeling free

Think of being able to enjoy a smorgasbord or a special dinner, or even just a snack, with no worries about calories or weight gain. Think of being able to eat just one chocolate and feel satisfied. Think of how good it would feel to decide on carrots rather than carrot cake because it was what you really wanted.

The long-term results are:

· A healthy body and mind
· A feeling of pleasure while you eat in moderation
· A feeling of freedom, of being a natural eater

If you decide to jump in with both feet, try saying to yourself The Nectar Pledge:

"This program is a way to fix the rest of my life so that I can live happily with food. It has taken me many years to reach this state. I have been practicing unnatural eating behaviors for so long, surely I can allow myself to slip now and then. It's not a disaster if I have a binge; my binges are shorter and happen less often. If I persevere with this new thinking, eventually I will not binge. I have been told that change will be slow. I can give myself at least two years to absorb thoroughly the idea that everybody chooses their behavior. This is a new way to think. The old way didn't work, and I can now choose a new, natural eating behavior."

Or, just say to yourself, "There's no rush. I can make it."

What is the cost of Nectar? Giving up the terror and fear of gaining weight, and the restrictions of dieting, that are associated with wanting to lose weight. When you compare this expectation to the statistics of how few people achieve weight loss by dieting, is it so much to give up?

Once you achieve a Nectar lifestyle you will be a natural eater, enjoying your freedom and your food. Food will no longer be a major focus in your life. Food will become just a normal, natural part of your existence, to be enjoyed when you are hungry. You will exercise not because you are chasing weight loss but because it feels good, and because your body feels energetic and healthy. Because you are using control theory in your life, you will find that you are more aware of meeting your needs, and will be better equipped to balance your life so that you can handle stress and relationships in more effective ways.

Nectar does not give you a simple prescription for what to do to achieve your new lifestyle. In fact, when you are truly using Nectar principles, you will feel as though you are doing nothing about your eating or your weight. You will feel as though you are eating as much as ever, and feel satisfied with how much and what you are eating. You will be able to go back to eating with the family, and will join in on the occasional feast without

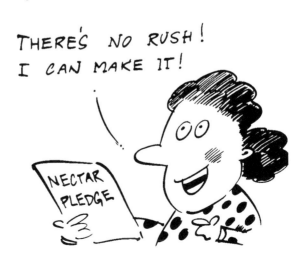

worrying about consequences. People who are still "thinking fat" will look at *you* and think, "It's not fair how much you eat and still look great!"

And you will give a sweet little smile and hand them this book.

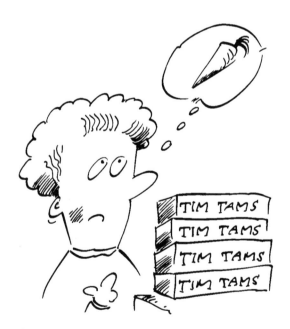

I'D GIVE ANYTHING FOR A CARROT !

RECOMMENDED READINGS

Atrens, Dale. *Don't Diet*. New York: Bantam, 1988.

Boffey, Barnes. *Reinventing Yourself*. Chapel Hill, NC: New View, 1993.

Covey, Stephen. *The Seven Habits of Highly Effective People*. New York: Simon and Schuster, 1989.

Ford, Edward E. *Choosing to Love*. Scottsdale, AZ: Brandt, 1987.

_____ . *Freedom from Stress*. Scottsdale, AZ: Brandt, 1989.

_____ . *Love Guaranteed*. Scottsdale, AZ: Brandt, 1987.

Glasser, William. *Control Theory*. New York: Harper Collins, 1984.

Good, E. Perry. *In Pursuit of Happiness*. Chapel Hill, NC: New View, 1987.

Hirshmann, Jane R., and Munter, Carol H. *Overcoming Overeating*. New York: Ballentine Books, 1988.

McFadden, Judy. *The Simple Way to Raise a Good Kid*. Cammeray, Australia: Horowitz Grahame. 1988.

NECTAR GROUPS

If you try out Nectar thinking on your own and begin to feel the freedom of these new ideas, but, like me, you need support, you could write New View for information about a Nectar group in your area. Pilot groups are now available in: Lubbock, Texas; Chapel Hill and Charlotte, North Carolina; Newport, Rhode Island; and Richmond, Virginia.

It was the group process that helped me to really "get" the whole picture. You do find out that your behaviors are not so awful, and that others have been through the same agonies as you. The Nectar group program contains many ideas and activities, in addition to those in this book, which help you to learn natural eating and applications of control theory. People comment on the fun, the learning and most important, the lack of criticism.

If there is no instructor in your area and you believe the demand is great, write New View and let them know. Perhaps you might think about learning to present the program yourself. Nectar group instructors are trained to understand both eating problems and human behavior, based on the specialized ideas of control theory. There are really three essentials that we have found make a good Nectar instructor: ability to teach information to adults, understanding control theory, and an understanding of eating problems. (Is this the first time that being fat has been an important qualification for a job?) It also helps to have a concern for people and a sense of humor, of course. If you want to apply for training, send your name to New View.

New View/Nectar America
P.O. Box 3021, Chapel Hill, NC 27515
919-942-8491